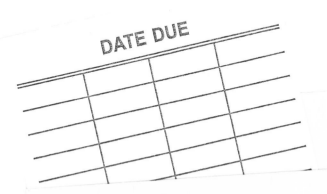

DATE DUE

Governors State University
Library
Hours:
Monday thru Thursday 8:30 to 10:30
Friday and Saturday 8:30 to 5:00
Sunday 1:00 to 5:00 (Fall and Winter Trimester Only)

DEMCO

The Brain and Sensory Plasticity:
Language Acquisition and Hearing

Edited by

**Charles I. Berlin, Ph.D.
and Theodore G. Weyand, Ph.D.**

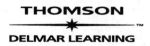

THOMSON

DELMAR LEARNING

Australia Canada Mexico Singapore Spain United Kingdom United States

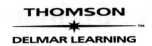

THOMSON

DELMAR LEARNING

The Brain and Sensory Plasticity: Language Acquisition and Hearing
Edited by
Charles I. Berlin and Theodore G. Weyand

Vice President,
Health Care Business Unit:
William Brottmiller

Editorial Director:
Cathy L. Esperti

Developmental Editor:
Maria D'Angelico

Marketing Director:
Jennifer McAvey

Editorial Assistant:
Chris Manion

Production Editor:
James Zayicek

Technology Specialist:
Victoria Moore

Library of Congress
Cataloging-in-Publication Data

The brain and sensory plasticity : language acquisition and hearing / edited by Charles I. Berlin, Theodore G. Weyand.
    p. cm.
    Includes bibliographical references and index.
    ISBN 1-4018-3947-9
    1. Auditory cortex. 2. Neuroplasticity. 3. Language acquisition. I. Berlin, Charles I. II. Weyand, Theodore Gordon.

QP383.15.B725 2003
152.1'5—dc21   2003041984

NOTICE TO THE READER

Publisher does not warrant or guarantee any of the products described herein or perform any independent analysis in connection with any of the product information contained herein. Publisher does not assume, and expressly disclaims, any obligation to obtain and include information other than that provided to it by the manufacturer.

The reader is expressly warned to consider and adopt all safety precautions that might be indicated by the activities described herein and to avoid all potential hazards. By following the instructions contained herein, the reader willingly assumes all risks in connection with such instructions.

The publisher makes no representations or warranties of any kind, including but not limited to, the warranties of fitness for particular purpose or merchantability, nor are any such representations implied with respect to the material set forth herein, and the publisher takes no responsibility with respect to such material. The publisher shall not be liable for any special, consequential, or exemplary damages resulting, in whole or part, from the reader's use of, or reliance upon, this material.

Contents

Contents

Preface

The Brain and Sensory Plasticity: Language Acquisition and Hearing is the eighth book in the Kresge-Mirmelstein Award cycle published and supported by Delmar Learning. The series was conceived by the late Rona Mirmelstein, a great benefactor of the Kresge Lab, and Dr. Charles Berlin. Mrs. Mirmelstein's daughter, Karyl Ann "Kam" Mirmelstein Lemberger, has also created a professorship at Kresge in her mother's name. Each year, the Kresge Lab gives a cash prize to a peer-selected scientist who made a singularly powerful and original contribution to hearing science. At the awarding of the prize, talks are presented, orchestrated around the prize winner's topic. The talks become chapters, and the chapters become books like this one. This book, the eighth in the series, celebrates Masakazu Konishi, who has led the field of neuroethology since the 1960s. Konishi's award was presented on October 8, 2001. He was selected to receive the prize by a truly august panel: the previous seven winners of the Kresge Mirmelstein award. They were Drs. Bill Brownell, Bob Wenthold, David Kemp, M. Charles Liberman, Karen Steele, David Corey, and Peter Dallos, all celebrated scientists in their field. We thank both Kam Mirmelstein Lemberger and Frances Barnes Bullington for their continued support of our efforts.

Charles I. Berlin, Ph.D.
Clinical Professor Otolaryngology, Head and Neck Surgery
Kenneth & Frances Barnes Bullington Professor of Hearing Science
Retired September 1, 2002 as Director of Kresge Hearing Research Laboratory

List of Contributors

Charles I. Berlin, Ph.D.
Kresge Hearing Research
  Laboratory
Louisiana State University
  Health Sciences Center
New Orleans, LA

Carmen C. Canavier, Ph.D.
Department of Psychology
University of New Orleans
New Orleans, Louisiana

William Guido
Kresge Hearing Research
  Laboratory
Department of Otolaryngology
Louisiana State University
  Health Sciences Center
New Orleans, Louisiana

Linda J. Hood, Ph.D.
Kresge Hearing Research
  Laboratory
Department of Otolaryngology
Louisiana State University
  Health Sciences Center
New Orleans, Louisiana

Masakazu Konishi, Ph.D.
Bing Professor of Behavioral
  Biology,
Division of Biology
California Institute of
  Technology
Pasadena, California

Fu-Sun Lo
Kresge Hearing Research
  Laboratory
Department of Otolaryngology
Louisiana State University
  Health Sciences Center
New Orleans, Louisiana

L.P. Lovejoy
M.D./Ph.D. program
University of California at San
  Diego
San Diego, California

Thierry Morlet, Ph.D.
Kresge Hearing Research
  Laboratory
Department of Otolaryngology
Louisiana State University
  Health Sciences Center
New Orleans, Louisiana

Michael Norman
University of Texas Academy
   of Distinguished Teachers
R.P. Doherty Professor of
   Communication
   University of Texas at
   Austin
Departments of Linguistics
   and Communication
   Sciences and Disorders
   Austin, Texas

Siva Perla
Department of Psychology
University of New Orleans
New Orleans, Louisiana

Beverly Ray
University of Texas Academy
   of Distinguished Teachers
R.P. Doherty Professor of
   Communication
   University of Texas at
   Austin
Departments of Linguistics
   and Communication
   Sciences and Disorders
   Austin, Texas

P. D. Shepard
Maryland Psychiatric Research
   Center
University of Maryland School
   of Medicine
Baltimore, Maryland

Harvey M. Sussman, Ph.D.
University of Texas Academy
   of Distinguished Teachers
R.P. Doherty Professor of
   Communication
   University of Texas at
   Austin
Departments of Linguistics
   and Communication
   Sciences and Disorders
   Austin, Texas

Theodore G. Weyand, Ph.D.
Department of Cell Biology
   and Anatomy
Louisiana State University
   Health Sciences Center
New Orleans, LA

Jokubas Ziburkus
Kresge Hearing Research
   Laboratory
Department of Otolaryngology
Louisiana State University
   Health Sciences Center
New Orleans, Louisiana

1

Synthesis of Neural Representation of Auditory Space in Barn Owls

Masakazu Konishi, Ph.D.
Division of Biology 216-76
California Institute of Technology
Pasadena, CA

The ultimate goal of auditory physiology is to explain auditory perception in terms of connections and signals between neurons. This aim requires the integration of neurophysiological, anatomical, and behavioral studies. Many neurons at all levels of brain organization may participate in perceptual events. Our ability to observe all these neurons at once is still limited despite recent advances in brain imaging techniques. Recording of one neuron or a "single unit" at a time has been the technique used in most vertebrate sensory neurophysiology. This approach would be quite useless, if sensory information were encoded only by spatial or temporal distributions of activity in an ensemble of neurons. Tapping a single neuron at a time tells little about how the whole ensemble encodes information. When single neurons respond selectively to particular stimuli such as color and sound frequency, we assume that these neurons convey information about these stimulus properties. The goal of single-unit neurophysiology is not to make a catalogue of neuronal response types but to carry out systematic survey of brain pathways in which neurons are selective for certain stimuli or stimulus features that are relevant to perception. For example, neurons in one pathway may be sensitive to stimulus features that are related to spatial locations. Such pathways are called information streams. Here, combination of neurophysiological and anatomical studies is essential. Search for information streams turned out to be a powerful approach in the study of brain mechanisms of sound localization in owls.

Behavioral studies are essential for finding out what constitutes information in particular perceptual tasks. For example, what physical cues do owls use to localize prey in the dark? If we know the cues, we can look for neurons that selectively respond to them. If and where the desirable neurons occur, however, is a critical problem. Auditory processing starts with encoding of frequency, amplitude, and phase in the inner ear. Successive brain centers extract from the coded data information necessary for the synthesis of representations of complex stimuli. According to this simple scenario, one could ascend the hierarchy from the ear to the highest center where relevant stimuli are represented. Yet few studies have succeeded in using this bottom-up approach to explain auditory perception, because the neural representations of percepts are hard to predict. Lower-order neurons may respond to different features of a complex stimulus, but we cannot predict how they are put together to represent the stimulus in terms of responses of single neurons. Proceeding from the highest center and descending the hierarchy or a top-down approach is also possible. Here, the discovery of higher-order neurons sensitive to behaviorally significant stimuli is a prerequisite. In the study of the barn owl's auditory system, we assumed that the owl's brain should contain neurons sensitive to the direction of sound sources, because owls localize sound accurately (Knudsen & Konishi, 1978). The discovery of such space-specific neurons in a higher center led to the pathways and processes for the synthesis of this selectivity (Konishi, Takahashi, Wagner, Sullivan, & Carr, 1988). This chapter describes the work as if it proceeded from lower to higher centers.

ACOUSTIC CUES FOR SOUND LOCALIZATION

Barn owls use the interaural time difference (ITD) for localization in azimuth or the horizontal plane and the interaural level difference (ILD) for elevation (Moiseff, 1989a; Moiseff & Konishi, 1981). When a sound signal reaches one ear before the other ear, an ITD results. The ITD varies systematically as a function of sound source directions. The maximal ITD experienced by the owl is about 160 μsec when sound propagates along the aural axis (Moiseff, 1989b). The differences in arrival time between the ears come in two forms: one is the disparity in the first wave of the signal, which is referred to as "onset time difference," and the other is the disparity in "ongoing time difference," which is the phase difference in tones or in spectral components of a complex signal. Barn owls can use only the ongoing time difference for localization in azimuth (Moiseff & Konishi, 1981). The ILD refers to the condition in which sound is louder in one ear than in the other. The head casts a shadow in the sound field, reducing sound level more in one ear than in the other. The effects of shadowing vary with the direction of sound propagation relative to the head. Owls do not have any external ear, but the feather ruff that surrounds their face serves as a sound collecting devise. The facial ruff consists of left and right halves that are separated by a tall ridge of feathers along the midline of the face. In barn owls, the left ear opening is located higher in the ruff than the right one (Payne, 1971). This asymmetry and other differences between the left and right halves of the ruff make the left and right ears more sensitive to sound coming from below and above eye level, respectively. This difference in the ear's directional sensitivity causes the ILD to vary as a function of sound elevation. Given a constant size of the head and sound collectors, shorter wavelengths and thus higher frequencies produce greater level differences than lower frequencies. The barn owl needs relatively high frequencies (5–8 kHz) for accurate localization in elevation (Knudsen, Blasdel, & Konishi, 1979; Knudsen & Konishi, 1979). Other owl species that can hear high frequencies show ear asymmetries, but the facial and aural structures involved differ between species (Volman & Konishi, 1990). Interaural asymmetries are rare in other animals, although Searle, Braida, Cuddy, and Davis (1975) suggested that interaural differences in the human pinna might facilitate sound localization.

The barn owl naturally turns its head in the direction of sound sources, allowing the accuracy of localization to be measured objectively (Knudsen et al., 1979). Early studies obtained a good linear relationship between ITD and the angle of head orientation in azimuth. The response of owls to ILD only indicated that the owls interpreted sounds louder in the left ear as "downwards" and those louder in the right ear as "upwards" (Moiseff, 1989b; Moiseff & Konishi, 1981). Recent studies use head-related transfer functions (HRTFs), which are derived from the signals recorded near the owl's eardrum as a function of source directions (Keller, Hartung, & Takahashi, 1998). Each source direction corresponds to a specific set of cue values that include ITD, ILD, and certain monaural parameters. Owls respond to HRTF by turning their heads in the direction represented by the signal as accurately as that broadcast from a speaker (Egnor, 2000). Different variables of HRTFs can be changed for the study of their roles in sound localization. For example, both ITD and ILD vary not only with source directions but also with frequency. The question is whether the frequency-dependent variations are necessary for accurate localization. Pogoniatz, Nelken, and Wagner (2001) showed that owls could localize HRTF signals in which ITD did not change with frequency. In elevation, there were small differences between the unchanged HRTF signals and those in which ILDs changed with frequency (Egnor, 2000; Poganiatz & Wagner, 2001).

PARALLEL PATHWAYS

The barn owl derives both interaural cues from the same high frequency signal. Its auditory system processes the two cues in separate pathways within the brain stem (Sullivan & Konishi, 1984; Takahashi, Moiseff, & Konishi, 1984) (Figure 1-1). Birds have two anatomically separate cochlear nuclei on each side, the nucleus angularis and the nucleus magnocellularis, and each primary auditory fiber divides into two collaterals, one innervating the nucleus angularis and the other the nucleus magnocellularis (Carr & Boudreau, 1991). The two pathways that start from the cochlear nuclei are anatomically separate until they converge in the inferior colliculus (Takahashi & Konishi, 1988a, 1988b). The route from the nucleus magnocellularis will be referred to as the time pathway and that from the nucleus angularis as the level pathway.

NEURAL ENCODING OF INTERAURAL TIME DIFFERENCES

Phase Locking

When the inner ear decomposes complex signals into their frequency components, it encodes the phase and amplitude of each spectral component. Phase is encoded by phase-locked spikes, which are action potentials that occur at or near a particular phase

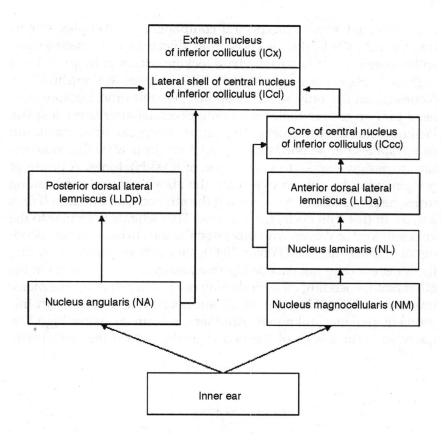

Figure 1-1. Parallel pathways. The owl's auditory system processes ITD and ILD in separate pathways that begin at the level of cochlear nuclei. The nucleus magnocellularis (NM) is the first station in the time pathway, and the nucleus angularis (NA) is the first station in the level pathway. The two routes unite in the inferior colliculus. Each primary auditory fiber from the inner ear divides into two branches of which one innervates the nucleus magnocellularis and the other the nucleus angularis. The nucleus laminaris (NL) is the first site where ITDs are detected. The nucleus laminaris projects to both the anterior dorsal lateral lemniscus (LLDa) and the core of the central nucleus of the inferior colliculus (ICcc). The core projects to the lateral shell of the central nucleus of the inferior colliculus (ICcl) on the contralateral side. The first site of ILD processing is the posterior dorsal lateral lemniscus (LLDp), which projects to the lateral shell of the central nucleus of the inferior colliculus. The ITD and ILD pathways merge without mixing different frequency bands in the lateral shell, which projects to the external nucleus of the inferior colliculus (ICx) where convergence across frequency occurs. Arrows indicate orthodoromic connections and the direction of information flow.

angle of tonal stimuli or spectral components of complex signals (Figure 1-2). Owls derive ITDs from disparities in phase-locked spikes between the two ears. Phase locking occurs at frequencies as high as 9 kHz in barn owls (Köppl, 1997; Sullivan & Konishi, 1984). Neurons can fire only so many spikes per unit time, because they need time to restore their membrane potential after firing a spike. We know that the owl's primary auditory fibers can fire a maximum of 800 spikes per second, which is a far cry from 8000 that is necessary to assign a spike to every cycle of 8000-Hz tones. A group of neurons may be able to overcome the above constraint by taking turns: neuron A fires a spike during the nth cycle, and neuron B fires a spike in $(n + 1)$th cycle, for example. This scheme is similar to the volley theory of Wever, who proposed the idea to explain the encoding of high frequencies (Wever, 1949), although we know today that the inner ear does not encode high frequency in this manner. On the other hand, encoding all periods may not be necessary for the measurement of ITDs. How the owl's auditory system deals with this problem remains unknown. Another problem in using high frequencies is the length of the period during which the cell's mem-

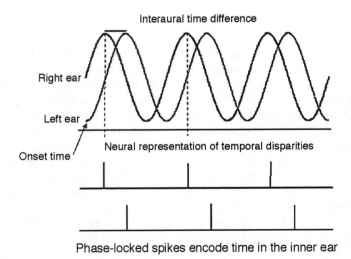

Figure 1-2. Neural representation of interaural temporal disparities. Neurons in the auditory nerve and those in the nucleus magnocellularis fire at or near a particular phase angle of tonal stimuli. This phenomenon is called phase locking. The owl derives ITDs from temporal disparities in phase-locked spikes between the ears.

brane potential changes, that is, action potential. This period is usually about 1 msec. Even if it is 0.5 msec, which is 500 μsec, it is still four times longer than a single period of 8000 Hz (125 μsec), meaning that four cycles of sound waves occur during a spike. What anatomical and physiological properties underlie fast responses in the time pathway is not known. Neurons of the nucleus magnocellularis in chicks, however, show a number of morphological and physiological adaptations for time coding such as end bulb–type terminals, nonlinear current-voltage relationships, and rapidly activating and slowly inactivating potassium currents (Trussell, 1999, for review). Similar morphological features in the owl's nucleus magnocellularis suggest fast-acting membrane mechanisms (Carr & Boudreau, 1991; see Carr & Friedman, 1999, for review).

Delay Lines and Coincidence Detection

Jeffress (1948) proposed a simple model for encoding ITDs for sound localization (Figure 1-3). The model consists of an array of neurons that receive input by systematically graded axonal paths

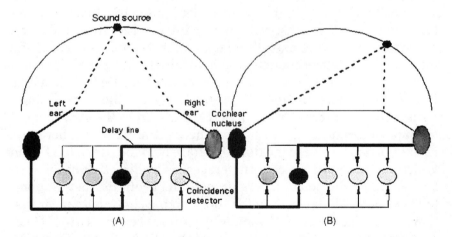

Figure 1-3. A model of delay line and coincidence detection. Coincidence detectors fire maximally when spikes from the two sides reach them simultaneously. A coincidence occurs when the sum of acoustic and neural transmission delays is equal for the two sides. The center coincidence detector fires when the sound source is directly in front (A). When the source moves toward the right ear, the acoustic delay for that side shortens. Thus, the site of coincidence detection in this array of neurons moves toward the cell that receives signals by a longer path from the right ear (B).

from the ipsi- and contralateral sides. The neurons act as coincidence detectors and fire maximally when spikes from the two sides arrive simultaneously. A coincidence occurs when the sum of acoustic and neural transmission delays on one side equals that on the other side, that is, $A_i + N_i = A_c + N_c$, where A indicates acoustic and N neural delays and subscripts i and c ipsilateral and contralateral, respectively. N_c and N_i vary systematically so as to accommodate all biologically relevant ITDs. Barn owls use a circuit and process similar to the above model to measure ITDs.

Neurons of the nucleus laminaris receive inputs from both the left and right magnocellular nuclei; thus, they are the first binaural neurons in the time pathway. Parks and Rubel (1975), finding similar connections in the chick's hind brain, suggested that these circuits could serve as delay lines and coincidence detectors in the measurement of ITDs as in the Jeffress model. In barn owls, anatomical studies and single neuron recordings from both the incoming magnocellular axons and laminaris neurons established that the axons work as delay lines and the neurons as coincidence detectors (Carr & Konishi, 1990) (Figure 1-4). In the chick's nucleus laminaris, the axons from the ipsilateral magnocellular nucleus are of equal length, whereas those from the contralateral side vary systematically in length. In the owl's nucleus laminaris, the magnocellular axons vary systematically in both ipsi- and contralateral sides.

Measurement of axonal delays within the nucleus laminaris indicates that delays change systematically from both the left and right entry points of the axons (Carr & Konishi, 1990). The axons from the ipsilateral magnocellular nucleus enter the nucleus laminaris from the dorsal surface, whereas those from the contralateral magnocellular nucleus enter from the ventral surface. Therefore, laminaris neurons near the dorsal surface must be tuned to ITDs in which the sound in the contralateral ear is leading that in the ipsilateral ear. As the position of neurons shifts ventrally, they respond to ITDs in which the lead by the sound in the contralateral ear systematically decreases. The laminaris neuron's selectivity for ITD is, therefore, mapped from dorsal to ventral (Peña, Viete, Funabiki, Saberi, & Konishi, 2001). Because the nucleus is divided into tonotopic bands, each band contains a map of ITDs.

Laminaris neurons are coincidence detectors and tuned to ITDs, yet they still respond to monaural stimuli from either side. Interestingly, they fire 1.5 times more spikes than the sum of left and right monaural spike rates in response, when the left and right

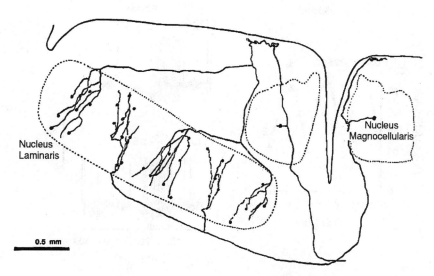

Figure 1-4. Nucleus laminaris. The nucleus laminaris receives input from both the left and right magnocelluar chochlear nuclei. Axons from the ipsilateral nucleus take circuitous courses to enter the nucleus laminaris from its dorsal surface, whereas those from the contralateral nucleus magnocellularis cross the midline to enter the nucleus laminaris from the ventral surface. The two population of axons course across the nucleus laminaris. It is this part of the axons that serves as delay lines. (From Carr & Konishi, 1990.)

inputs arrive simultaenously, whereas the spike rate is less than the mean of the monaural rates, when the left and right inputs arrive 180 degrees apart (Peña, Viete, Albeck, & Konishi, 1996). These findings suggest that laminaris neurons multiply inputs from the two sides.

Phase Ambiguity

Neurons of the nucleus laminaris and the medial superior olive respond to an ITD and ITD $\pm nT$, where n is an integer and T is the period of the stimulus tone (Carr & Konishi, 1990; Goldberg & Brown, 1969; Peña et al., 1996; Viete, Peña, & Konishi, 1997; Yin & Chan, 1990) (Figure 1-5). This phenomenon is referred to as phase ambiguity in the owl literature and "cyclic" in the mammalian literature. The neurons are responding to the interaural phase difference, which does not change by addition or subtraction of nT. The phenomenon can also be explained in terms of phase-locked

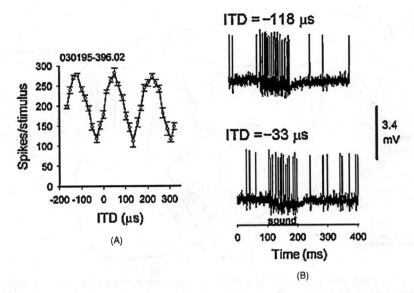

Figure 1-5. Phase ambiguity. Nucleus laminaris neurons are tuned to an ITD and its phase equivalents (ITD ± T, where T is the period of the stimulus tone). The response of a neuron to multiple ITDs is referred to as phase ambiguity. (From Peña et al., 1996.) Part B shows the response of a single neuron to ITDs conveyed by 5.9-kHz (T = 169 μsec) tones. ITD = –118 msec (tone in the left ear leading that in the right ear) induced a maximal rate of discharge and ITD = –33 a minimal rate. The stimulus tone lasted from 100 to 200 msec on the horizontal time axis. The spikes outside this range are spontaneous discharge. Part A shows an ITD curve in which the spike rates are plotted against ITD. The three peaks occur at –118 msec, +51 msec (i.e., –118 + 169), and 220 msec (i.e., –118 + 2 x 169).

spikes. In the simplest case, consecutive phase-locked spikes are separated by the tonal period (T). Suppose setting the ITD to a specific value ITDi causes two such trains to coincide spike by spike. Starting from this state, the two trains coincide again every time one train is either advanced or delayed by T. This explanation is another way of saying that the two trains coincide when they are separated by temporal disparities of ITDi or ITDi ± nT. ITDi is defined as the ITD to which a neuron responds with an equal spike rate independent of frequency and referred to the characteristic delay (Rose, Gross, Geisler, & Hind,1966). Yin and Chan (1990) developed a quantitative method to derive the ITDi from a neuron's ITD response curves obtained for different frequencies.

Resolution of Phase Ambiguity

The owl's brain derives the characteristic delay from ITD data coming from different frequency bands. Laminaris neurons project to two higher-order stations, the core of the central nucleus of the inferior colliculus (ICcc) and the anterior dorsal lateral lemniscus (LLDa). The ICcc projects to the lateral shell of the central nucleus (ICcl) of the inferior colliculus on the opposite hemisphere. All these areas are tonotopically organized so that ITD sensitivity is transmitted in each frequency band separately. ICcl projects to the external nucleus of the inferior colliculus (ICx). Here neurons tuned to different frequencies converge on single ICx neurons. These cells respond to ITDs like laminaris neurons when the stimulus is narrowband. In contrast, when the stimulus is broadband, ICx neurons respond best to the ITDi and not at all or much less to ITD$i \pm nT$, where T is now the inverse of the best frequency of the neuron. The peak at the ITDi is referred to as the main peak and peaks at ITD$i \pm nT$ side peaks. When the side peaks are smaller than the main peak, the phenomenon is referred to as side-peak suppression, although the size difference is mainly due to the facilitation of the main peak (Arthur, 2002; Mazer, 1998).

We proposed a model to account for side-peak suppression (Konishi et al., 1988; Wagner, Takahashi, & Konishi, 1987). An ICx neuron receives inputs from neurons selective for the same ITDi but tuned to different frequencies (Figure 1-6). Addition of these inputs across frequencies should give rise to a large peak at the ITDi and smaller peaks at ITD$i \pm nT$. Because T varies with frequency, mismatches in the side peaks emerge as shown in Figure 1-7. Trahiotis and Stern (1994) proposed a similar model to explain why humans localize narrowband signals ambiguously and broadband signals unambiguously. Note that there is a single straight line at ITDi and curved lines connecting ITD$i \pm nT$. These authors argued that humans evaluate the straightness of the curve to discriminate between the ITDi and ITD$i \pm nT$.

We understand how the model works at the level of single neurons. Single ICx neurons receive inputs from ICcl neurons that are tuned to the same ITDi but to different frequencies as in Figure 1-7. Intracellular recordings allow us to see these inputs in terms of postsynaptic potentials (PSPs). The main ITD peak is

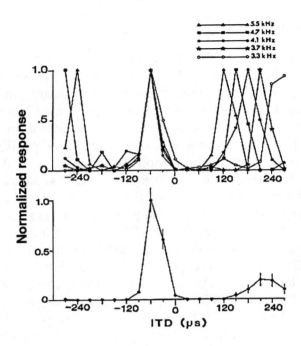

Figure 1-6. Frequency convergence and ITD responses. ICx neurons like the one in this figure respond to multiple ITDs when stimulated with tones (upper panel). Note that there is one peak where all curves converge, which is the main peak at the ITD*i*. The position of side peaks varies between 120 and 240 µsec according to the stimulus frequency. The same neuron responds to a broadband signal with one peak at the ITD*i* (lower panel).

only slightly taller than the side peaks in these PSPs (Peña & Konishi, 2000). PSPs give rise to spikes when they cross the threshold of spike discharge. The main peak is much taller than the side peaks in the ITD curve of spike rates. This difference between the PSP and spike rate ITD curves is attributable to thresholding (Albeck & Konishi, 1995; Peña & Konishi, 2002). When the spike threshold occurs below the tip of the main peak but above that of the side peaks, the neuron will have a single ITD peak at ITD*i*. Although this situation does occur for some ICx neurons, for the majority the spike threshold is well below the main peak but only slightly below the tips of the side peaks. This condition gives rise to a tall main peak and smaller side peaks in spike rates. We do not know, however, whether and how the spike threshold is adjusted to discriminate between the ITD peaks.

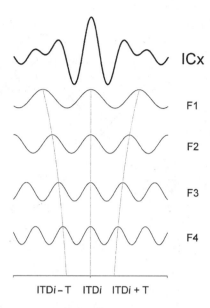

ITD*i* – T   ITD*i*   ITD*i* + T

Figure 1-7. Resolution of phase ambiguity. The observations in Figure 1-6 led to a model for resolving the phase ambiguity. The ICx neuron receives ITD information from different frequency bands (F1, F2, etc.). The straight line connecting the ITD curves of different frequencies indicates the frequency independent ITD*i*. Note that addition of ITD responses across frequency gives rise to a tall peak at the ITD*i* (thick curve) and smaller peaks at other ITDs.

NEURAL ENCODING
OF INTERAURAL LEVEL DIFFERENCES

The first binaural station in the level pathway is the posterior dorsal lateral lemniscus (LLDp) that receives a direct excitatory input from the contralateral nucleus angularis and an inhibitory input from the LLDp of the opposite side (Adolphs, 1993; Takahashi & Keller, 1992) (Figure 1-8). Stimulation of the contralateral ear excites LLDp neurons almost as a linear function of sound level, and sound in the ipsilateral ear inhibits them. The more intense the sound, the stronger the inhibition. Thus, the response of LLDp neurons varies as a function of sound levels in the two ears, that is, ILD. Stimulation with ILD gives rise to a sigmoidal curve that starts from a high spike rate for contralateral stimulation and ends with a low rate for ipsilateral stimulation. Furthermore, both the threshold and the strength of inhibition change from dorsal to ventral in this nucleus. This gradient gives rise to a map of ILD in

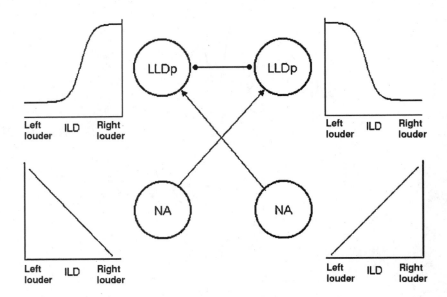

Figure 1-8. Circuits for creating sensitivity to ILD. The first site where sensitivity to ILD emerges is LLDp. In this idealized model, the response of NA neurons varies linearly with sound level. LLDp neurons show a sigmoidal response curve to ILD, because excitation from the contralateral NA and inhibition from the contralateral LLDp interact. Both the threshold and degree of inhibition vary systematically within the nucleus, indicating a map of ILD sensitivity within the nucleus.

which neurons more sensitive to contralateral sound occur dorsally and those that prefer equal sound level in both ears ventrally (Manley, Köppl, & Konishi, 1988; Mogdans & Knudsen, 1994; Takahashi, Barberini, & Keller, 1995). These neurons are not perfect detectors of ILD, however, because monaural stimuli from the contralateral ear alone can drive them. Neurons that require exclusively binaural stimuli emerge in the ICx and this property is attributable to inhibition induced by ILDs that depart far from the neuron's best ILD (Adolphs, 1993; Peña & Konishi, 2002).

CONVERGENCE OF ITD AND ILD PATHWAYS

The nucleus laminaris projects to LLDa and the core of the central nucleus of the inferior colliculus (ICcc) (see Figure 1-1). Core neurons then project to the lateral shell of the central nucleus of the inferior colliculus (ICcl) on the contralateral side. LLDp projects to the lateral shell of both sides. Therefore, the two pathways converge in the lateral shell. This area is tonotopically organized, indicating that

ITD and ILD sensitive neurons are frequency tuned. The lateral shell projects to the adjoining external nucleus of the inferior colliculus (ICx) where neurons tuned to different frequencies converge. ICx neurons are broadly frequency-tuned and sensitive to combinations of ITD and ILD. ICx neurons respond only to signals coming from particular directions, because they are selective for specific combinations of ITD and ILD. Figure 1-9 shows what the combination

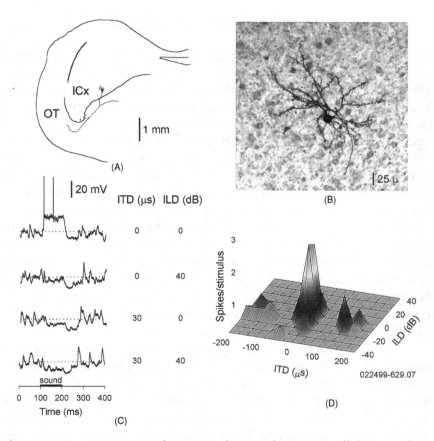

Figure 1-9. Sensitivity to combinations of ITD and ILD. Intracellular recordings show that favorable combinations of ITD and ILD induce excitatory postsynaptic potentials (EPSPs) and unfavorable ones, either inhibitory postsynaptic potentials (IPSPs) or subthreshold membrane potentials created by the mixture of EPSP and IPSP. (A) A camera lucida drawing of ICx, which is surrounded by the optic tectum (OT). (B) A photomicrograph of the ICx neuron used in this experiment. (C) Sample subthreshold (membrane) responses of the neurons to different combinations of ITD and ILD. The dotted line indicates the resting membrane potential. (D) Sub- and suprathreshold esponses of the same neuron to a large number of ITD-ILD pairs. (From Peña & Konishi, 2001.)

sensitivity means in terms of membrane potentials. This neuron responded best to the combination (ITD = 0, ILD = 0) as seen in the amplitude of excitatory postsynaptic potential. The membrane potential remained below threshold (dotted line) for other combinations, including (0, 40), (30, 0) and (30, 40). We now know that the combination sensitivity is due to multiplication of postsynaptic potentials for ITD and ILD (Peña & Konishi, 2001).

A MAP OF AUDITORY SPACE

ICx neurons have spatial receptive fields, because they are tuned to combinations of ITD and ILD, which encode auditory space (Figure 1-10). The idea that auditory space may be mapped in the brain goes back to Jeffress's classical paper entitled "A place theory of sound localization," although this paper is better known for the concept of delay lines and coincidence detection (Jeffress, 1948). Neither the pattern nor the rate of spikes but the place of coincidence detectors in the circuit codes for the azimuthal direction of sound sources. We did not know this idea when we started to look for a map of auditory space in the owl's auditory system. Starr (1974) argued that neither spatial receptive fields nor maps of space should exist in the auditory system, because space is not mapped in the sensory surface as in the visual and somatosensory systems. Brain maps that result from topographical projections of sensory surface are referred to as projection maps, in contrast with computational maps that are centrally synthesized (Knudsen, Du Lac, & Esterly, 1987; Konishi, 1986).

The space map projects to the optic tectum to form a bimodal map of space (Knudsen & Knudsen, 1983). Thus, the computational map is created so that a single spatial coordinate system may be used for the two different sensory modalities (Knudsen & Brainard, 1995). Barn owl use head-centered coordinates for both auditory and visual space. Thus, when the head moves, the coordinate centers for both modalities move with the head. The owl turns its head to see and hear objects in space, because the owl can move neither its eyes nor its ears (unlike the mammalian pinna). Thus, the owl need not adjust the neural representation of auditory space in response to gaze shifts. If bimodal neurons' visual receptive fields are shifted by prisms, however, the auditory receptive fields gradually change in the direction of the visual ones (see Knudsen, 2002, for review). Such adjustments occur not only in

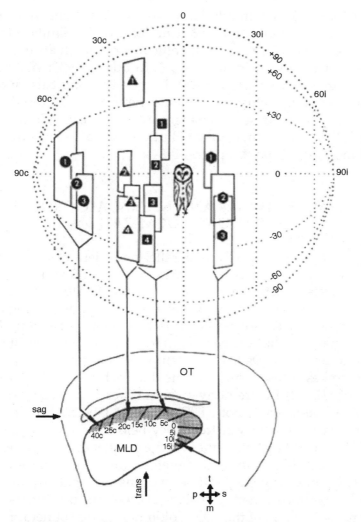

Figure 1-10. A map of auditory space. The sensitivity for combinations of ITD and ILD underlies the formation of spatial receptive fields by space-specific neurons. Because space is not encoded in the inner ear, the auditory system produces space maps by computation. Each rectangle indicates the center of a neuron's receptive field in real space. The numbers indicate the sequence in which the neurons were recorded during one electrode penetration. Negative – and positive + signs show below and above eye level, respectively. Notations 90i, 90c, and so forth indicate spatial angles on the ipsi (i) and contralateral (c) side with respect to the side of the brain in which the map occurs. The map represents the contralateral hemifield with a small extension into the ipsilateral field. The bottom panel shows a section across the optic lobe. MLD is the avian term for the inferior colliculus. The shaded area is the ICx. Arrows show the relationships between the anatomical locations of neurons and their receptive fields in space. Notations 5i, 5c, and so forth denote the spatial angles mapped. (From Knudsen & Konishi, 1978.)

young owls but also in adults, if visual shifts occur in an incremental manner (Linkenhoker & Knudsen, 2002). Similar bimodal maps are found in the superior colliculus of mammals (e.g., King & Hutchings, 1984; Middlebrooks & Knudsen, 1987; Withington, Binns, Ingham, & Thorton, 1994). In monkeys and cats, auditory spatial receptive fields of collicular neurons shift rapidly and reversibly in response to changes in gaze (e.g., Groh, Tause, Underhill, Clark, & Inati, 2001; Hartline, Vimal, King, Kurylo, & Northmore, 1995); Jay & Sparks, 1984).

BRAIN NETWORK AND NEURAL ALGORITHM FOR SOUND LOCALIZATION

Figure 1-11 summarizes how parallel and hierarchical networks synthesize the selectivity for combinations of ITD and ILD. Many sensory systems separate different aspects of natural stimuli and process them in separate pathways. Hierarchical processing is also common in most sensory systems and an important aspect of code transformation. The nucleus laminaris creates "labeled lines" or "place codes" for ITDs from the temporal codes carried by phase-locked spikes. These terms indicate that each neuron is tuned to a range of ITDs. ILDs are derived from differences in sound levels and also line-labeled. Both ITD and ILD labeled lines are also tuned to narrow bands of frequency below the level of the ICcl. The ITD and ILD labeled lines merge frequency by frequency in the ICcl. Each ICcl neuron is, therefore, tuned to a specific set of ITD, ILD, and frequency. These neurons are spatially arranged such that neurons tuned to specific ITDs occur in columns across the tonotopic layers of the ICcl. Columnar groups of neurons project to single ICx neurons. The convergence of ICcl neurons across different frequencies leads to broad frequency tuning in ICx neurons. As a result, the ICx does not contain a map of frequency but a map of auditory space. ICx neurons represent the results of all computations that take place in the pathways leading to them and those that they perform by themselves.

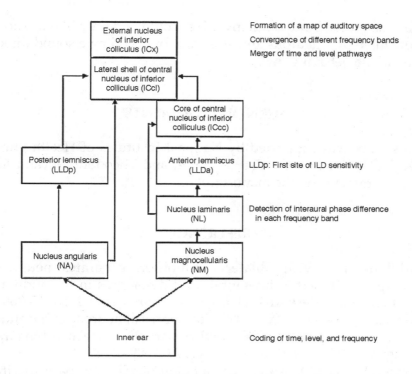

Figure 1-11. Neural network and algorithm. This figure summarizes the successive stages of signal processing and synthesis leading to the selectivity of space-specific neurons for space. It shows how the owl's auditory system creates neuronal selectivity for auditory space and confers it on single neurons at the top of parallel hierarchically organized neural networks.

CONCLUSIONS

Recent papers argue whether the auditory system uses place or ensemble coding for space. For example, McAlpine, Jiang, and Palmer (2001) and Schnupp (2000) assume that the owl's auditory system uses place coding. Place or labeled-line coding uses a single neuron to encode a particular source direction. Ensemble coding in its purest form would use a group of neurons that are not selective for any direction. The spatial and temporal distributions of activities within the ensemble can encode source directions. What those authors mean is a population of neurons that are broadly tuned to space. As long as the neurons are selective for stimuli, whether narrowly or broadly, they constitute labeled lines. In this sense, the distinction between the two schemes of coding is not qualitative but quantitative. We would certainly like to know how many ICx neurons are necessary for encoding a sound direction in the behaving owl.

ACKNOWLEDGMENTS

This work was supported by National Institutes of Health grant DC00134. I thank Drs. Charles Berlin and Theodore Weyand for their comments on the manuscript.

REFERENCES

Adolphs, R. (1993). Bilateral inhibition generates neuronal responses tuned to interaural level differences in the auditory brainstem of the barn owl. *Journal of Neuroscience, 13*, 3647–3668.

Albeck, Y., & Konishi, M. (1995). Responses of neurons in the auditory pathways of the barn owl to partially correlated binaural signals. *Journal of Neurophysiology, 74*, 1689–1700.

Arthur, B. J. (2002). Neural computations leading to space-specific auditory responses in the barn owl. Unpublished doctoral dissertation, California Institute of Technology.

Carr, C. E., & Boudreau, R. E. (1991). Central projections of auditory nerve fibers in the barn owl. *Journal of Comparative Neurology, 314*, 306–318.

Carr, C. E., & Friedman, M. A. (1999). Evolution of time coding systems. *Neural Computation, 11*, 1–20.

Carr, C. E., & Konishi, M. (1990). A circuit for detection of interaural time differences in the brainstem of the barn owl. *Journal of Neuroscience, 10*, 3227–3246.

Egnor, S. E. R. (2000). The role of spectral cues in sound localization by the barn owl. Unpublished doctoral dissertation, California Institute of Technology.

Goldberg, J. M., & Brown, P. B. (1969). Responses of binaual neurons of dog superio livary complex to dichotic tonal stimuli: Some physiological mechanisms of sound localization. *Journal of Neurophysiology, 32*, 613–636.

Groh, J. M., Trause, A. S., Underhill A. M., Clark K. R.,, & Inati, S. (2001). Eye position influences auditory responses in primate inferior colliculus. *Neuron, 29*, 509–518.

Hartline P. H., Vimal, R. L., King, A. J., Kurylo, D. D., & Northmore, D. P. (1995). Effects of eye position on auditory localization and neural representation of space in superior colliculus of cats. *Experimental Brain Research, 104*, 402–408.

Jay, M., & Sparks, D. (1984). Auditory receptive fields in primate superior colliculus shift with changes in eye position. *Nature, 309*, 345–347.

Jeffress, L. A. (1948). A place theory of sound localization. *Journal of Comparative and Physiological Psychology, 41*, 35–39.

Keller, C. H., Hartung, K., & Takahashi, T. T. (1998). Head-related transfer functions of the barn owl: Measurement and neural responses. *Hearing Research, 118*, 13–34.

King, A. J., & Hutchings, M. E. (1987). Spatial response properties of acoustically responsive neurons in the superior colliculus of the ferret: A map of auditory space. *Journal of Neurophysiology, 57*, 596–625.

Knudsen, E. I. (2002). Instructed learning in the auditory localization pathway of the barn owl. *Nature, 417*, 322–328.

Knudsen, E. I., Blasdel, G. G., & Konishi, M. (1979). Sound localization by the barn owl (*Tyto alba*) measured with the search coil technique. *Journal of Comparative Physiology, 133*, 1–11.

Knudsen E. I., & Brainard, M. S. (1995). Creating a unified representation of visual and auditory space in the brain. *Annual Review of Neuroscience, 18*, 19–14.

Knudsen, E. I., Du Lac, S., & Esterly, S. D. (1987). Computational maps in the brain. *Annual Review of Neuroscience, 10*, 41–65.

Knudsen, E. I., & Knudsen, P. F. (1983). Space-mapped auditory projections from the inferior colliculus to the optic tectum in the barn owl (*Tyto alba*). *Journal of Comparative Neurology, 218*, 187–196.

Knudsen, E. I., & Konishi, M. (1978). A neural map of auditory space in the owl. *Science, 200*, 795–797.

Knudsen, E. I., & Konishi, M. (1979). Mechanisms of sound localization in the barn owl (*Tyto alba*). *Journal of Comparative Physiology, 133*, 13–21.

Konishi, M. (1986). Centrally synthesized maps of sensory space. *Trends in Neurosciences, 9*, 163–168.

Konishi, M., Takahashi, T. T., Wagner, H., Sullivan, W. E., & Carr, C. E. (1988). Neurophysiological and anatomical substrates of sound localization in the owl. In G. M. Edelman, W. F. Wall, & W. M. Cowam (Eds.), *Auditory function* (pp. 721–745). New York: Wiley.

Köppl, C. (1997). Phase locking to high frequencies in the auditory nerve and cochlear nucleus magnocellularis of the barn owl, *Tyto alba. Journal of Neuroscience, 17,* 3312–3321.

Linkenhoker, B. A., & Knudsen, E. I. (2002). Incremental training increases the plasticity of the auditory space map in adult barn owls. *Nature, 419,* 293–296.

Manley, G. A., Köppl, C., & Konishi, M. (1988). A neural map of interaural intensity difference in the brainstem of the barn owl. *The Journal of Neuroscience, 8,* 2665–2676.

Mazer, J. A. (1998). How the owl resolves auditory coding ambiguity. *Proceedings of the National Academy of Sciences (USA), 95,* 10932–10937.

McAlpine, D., Jiang, D., & Palmer, A. R. (2001). A neural code for low-frequency sound localization in mammals. *Nature Neuroscience, 4,* 396–401.

Middlebrooks, J. C., & Knudsen, E. I. (1984). A neural code for auditory space in the cat's superior colliculus. *Journal of Neuroscience, 10,* 2621–2634.

Mogdans, J., & Knudsen, E. I. (1994). Representation of interaural level difference in the VLVp, the first site of binaural comparison in the barn owl's auditory system. *Hearing Research, 74,* 148–164.

Moiseff, A. (1989a). Bi-coordinate sound localization by the barn owl. *Journal of Comparative Physiology [A], 164,* 637–644.

Moiseff, A. (1989b). Binaural disparity cues available to the barn owl for sound localization. *Journal of Comparative Physiology [A], 164,* 629–636.

Moiseff, A., & Konishi, M. (1981). Neuronal and behavioral sensitivity to binaural time difference in the owl. *Journal of Neuroscience, 1,* 40–48.

Parks, T. N., & Rubel, E. W. (1975). Organization and development of brain stem auditory nuclei of the chicken: Organization of projections from n. magnocellularis to n. laminaris. *Journal of Comparative Neurology, 164,* 435–448.

Payne, R. S. (1971). Acoustic location of prey by barn owls (*Tyto alba*). *Journal of Experimental Biology, 54,* 535–573.

Peña, J. L., & Konishi, M. (2000). Cellular mechanisms for resolving phase ambiguity in the owl's inferior colliculus. *Proceedings of the National Academy of Sciences, 97,* 11787–11792.

Peña, J. L., & Konishi, M. (2001). Auditory spatial receptive fields created by multiplication. *Science, 292,* 249–252.

Peña, J. L., & Konishi, M. (2002). From postsynaptic potentials to spikes in the genesis of auditory spatial receptive fields. *Journal of Neuroscience, 22*, 5652–5658.

Peña, J. L., Viete, S., Albeck, Y., & Konishi, M. (1996). Tolerance to intense sound of binaural coincidence detection in the owl's nucleus laminaris. *Journal of Neuroscience, 16*, 7046–7054.

Peña, J. L., Viete, S. M., Funabiki, K., Saberi, K., & Konishi, M. (2001). Cochlear and neural delays for coincidence detection in owls. *Journal of Neuroscience, 21*, 9455–9459.

Poganiatz, I., Nelken, I., & Wagner, H. (2001). Sound-localization experiments with barn owls in virtual space: Influence of interaural time difference on head-turning behavior. *Journal of the Association for Research in Otolaryngology, 2*, 1–21.

Poganiatz, I., & Wagner, H. (2001). Sound-localization experiments with barn owls in virtual space: Influence of broadband interaural level difference on head-turning behavior. *Journal of Comparative Physiology [A], 187*, 225–233.

Rose, J. E., Gross, N. B., Geisler, C. D., & Hind, J. E. (1966). Some neural mechanisms in the inferior colliculus of the cat which may be relevant to localization of a sound source. *Journal of Neurophysiology, 29*, 288–314.

Schnupp, J. W. (2000). Of delays, coincidences and efficient coding for space in the auditory pathway. *Trends in Neurosciences, 24*, 677–678.

Searle, C. L., Braida, L. D., Cuddy, D. R., & Davis, M. F. (1975). Binaural pinna disparity: Another auditory localization cue. *Journal of the Acoustical Society of America, 57*, 448–455.

Starr, A. (1974). Neurophysiological mechanisms of sound localization. *Federation Proceedings, 33*, 1911–1914.

Sullivan, W. E., & Konishi, M. (1984). Segregation of stimulus phase and intensity in the cochlear nuclei of the barn owl. *Journal of Neuroscience, 4*, 1787–1799.

Takahashi, T. T., Barberini, C. L., & Keller, C. H. (1995). An anatomical substrate for the inhibitory gradient in the VL Vp of the owl. *Journal of Comparative Neurology, 358*, 294–304.

Takahashi, T. T., & Keller, C. H. (1992). Commisural connections mediate inhibition for the computation of interaural level difference in the barn owl. *Journal of Comparative Physiology [A], 170*, 161–169.

Takahashi, T. T., & Konishi, M. (1986). Selectivity for interaural time difference in the owl's midbrain. *Journal of Neuroscience, 6*, 3413–3422.

Takahashi, T. T., & Konishi, M. (1988a). Projections of nucleus angularis and nucleus laminaris to the lateral lemniscal nuclear complex of the barn owl. *Journal of Comparative Neurology, 274,* 212–238.

Takahashi, T. T., & Konishi, M. (1988b). Projections of the cochlear nuclei and nucleus laminaris to the inferior colliculus of the barn owl. *Journal of Comparative Neurology, 274,* 190–211.

Takahashi, T., Moiseff, A., & Konishi, M. (1984). Time and intensity cues are processed independently in the auditory system of the owl. *Journal of Neuroscience, 4,* 1781–1786.

Trahiotis, C., & Stern, R. M. (1994). Across-frequency integration in lateralization of complex binaural stimuli. *The Journal of the Acoustical Society of America, 96,* 3804–3806.

Trussell, L. O. (1999). Synaptic mechanisms for coding timing in auditory neurons. *Annual Review of Physiology, 61,* 477–496.

Viete, S., Peña, J. L., & Konishi, M. (1997). Effects of interaural intensity difference on the processing of interaural time difference in the owl's nucleus laminaris. *Journal of Neuroscience, 17,* 1815–1824.

Volman, S. F., & Konishi, M. (1990). Comparative physiology of sound localization in four species of owls. *Brain, Behavior and Evolution, 36,* 196–215.

Wagner, H., Takahashi, T. T., & Konishi, M. (1987). Representation of interaural time difference in the central nucleus of the barn owl's Inferior colliculus. *Journal of Neuroscience, 7,* 3105–3116.

Wever, E. G. (1949). *Theory of hearing.* New York: Wiley.

Withington, D. J., Binns, K. E., Ingham, N. J., & Thorton, S. K. (1994). Plasticity in the superior collicular auditory space map of adult guinea-pigs. *Experimental Physiology, 79,* 319–325.

Yin, T. C. T., & Chan, J. C. K. (1990). Interaural time sensitivity in medial superior olive of cat. *Journal of Neurophysiology, 64,* 465–488.

2

Neuroethology: Providing Insights Into Human Language Representation

Harvey M. Sussman, Ph.D.
Departments of Linguistics and Communication Sciences and Disorders
University of Texas at Austin
Austin, TX

An important challenge for cognitive neuroscience is to provide an understanding of *how* the brain accomplishes language. All too often the *where* component dominates scholarly publications as advances in brain imaging techniques far exceed our theoretical understanding of neural correlates of language. A first step in establishing a viable interface between language and the brain is compatibility between the nature of the stimuli being studied in the two domains. Language-based data should resemble neurophysiological data. At present, establishing explicit neural correlates for syntax and semantics is not feasible. This research focuses on a level of language organization that is compatible with data emanating from neurophysiological laboratories studying sensory processing in the brain of animal species. Specifically, this chapter describes how phonological categories are formed and how they might be encoded within neural substrates. The phonological level of human language structure is a form of human neuroethology. The strategy adopted here uses well-documented algorithms from neuroethology as theoretical springboards to help understand specific aspects of human auditory processing of speech. Two species that are biologically specialized for processing sounds—the barn owl and the bat—are particularly valuable in the study of sound encoding for human language. In addition, understanding how the visual system resolves decoding problems can also provide insights into human auditory perception and representation.

The rationale for using an animal-to-human approach is well founded. To begin with, the brain is a product of evolution, with a successful design and architecture already in place. Second, evolution tends to have similar solutions for similar problems. The lack of a common phyletic history across species does not preclude making generalizations from animal-to-human signal processing. Rather than forming an argument based on homology (Campbell, 1988), one can base the argument on homoplasy (Hodos, 1988), which "typically arises because even distantly related species will confront environmental problems with a limited set of adaptive solutions" (Hauser, 1996, p. 13). Last, there are more similarities than differences in the structure and function of auditory systems across species with common stimulus-processing requirements.

This chapter illustrates how a language-neuroethology link can be established. The focus is on a specific conundrum in speech production/perception known as the "noninvariance" problem. After a description of the problem and a possible phonetic-based solution, discussion turns to how the phonetic data from human speech parallels neuroethology data relating to how the barn owl's auditory processing system successfully resolves ambiguity in the input signal during the localization of sound. The crux of the processing problem faced by both the barn owl in sound localization and the human listener in categorizing stop consonants is to normalize the inherent variability of the input signal and thereby enable equivalence classes to form in a self-organizing and emergent fashion. The objective of this chapter is to describe such a process: one is well documented (barn owl), and the other is understandably speculative (human).

THE NONINVARIANCE PROBLEM IN SPEECH PERCEPTION

For over five decades speech scientists have struggled to explain how stop consonant + vowel utterances are categorized. To illustrate the nature of this sorting problem, consider the following: a listener hears the spoken words *"deet, debt, dit, date, dote, dot, doot, daught."* If you ask the listener what the initial sound was in each of the words, he or she would report a "d."

Not surprisingly, all the initial sounds are clearly perceived as a /d/, which does not sound terribly perplexing until one realizes that the physical sound structure of each word above is different. The vowels that follow the /d/ are different in each word. It is the "blending" of the consonant (C) and vowel (V) together that creates the physical differences in the speech signal that reaches the ear of the listener and becomes transformed into the neural signal under analysis for perceptual processing. Thus, the dilemma facing speech scientists is how to explain that a speech signal that is physically variable in each instance is nevertheless perceived as the same. The technical phrase used to describe this problem is acoustic variance and perceptual invariance.

To illustrate this phenomenon, examine the spectral composition of various words beginning with /d/ + vowel (V) sequences as illustrated in Figure 2-1. The speech spectrograms show the first (F1) and second (F2) formants of [dV] utterances spoken by an adult male speaker. Time is represented along the abscissa and frequency (Hz) along the ordinate. The top row, reading from left to right, displays [di] as in "deed," [dE] as in "dead," [dQ] as in "dad," and [do] as in "dough"; the bottom row shows [d'] as in "dumb," [da] as in "dot," [de] as in "day," and [du] as in "dew." The crucial portion to view is the initial part of F2, the transition, because this FM signal captures the changing resonance pattern of the vocal tract that directly reflects the moving tongue as it releases the occlusion for the stop and moves into position to shape the upcoming vowel. It can be seen that each [dV] utterance has a unique F2 transition depending on the ensuing vowel context. Transitions into vowels like /i/ and /e/ (e.g., "deet" and "day") go up in frequency, transitions into vowels like /o/ and /u/ ("dough" and "dew") move down in frequency. In essence, the upcoming vowel "colors" the articulatory patterns for the consonant, because the tongue anticipates the vowel during the consonantal gesture. All stop consonant categories (/bdgptk/) across the world's languages reflect this vowel-context-induced variability of the F2 transition. This perceptual enigma has been known for a long time (Liberman, Delattre, Cooper, & Gerstman, 1954), has instigated many decades of research, and has inspired many diverse perceptual theories, yet a satisfactory empirical and theoretical resolution has remained elusive.

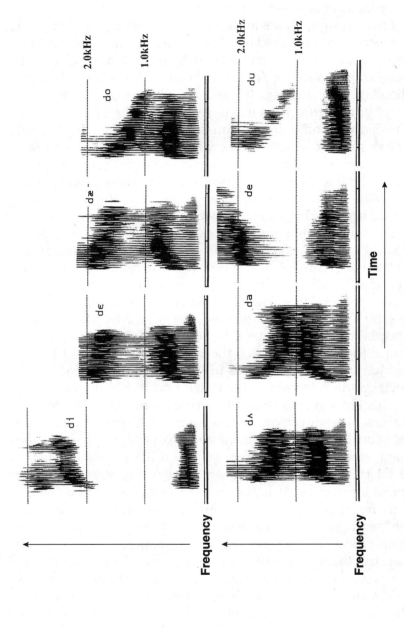

Figure 2-1. Speech spectrograms of initial consonant /d/ + vowel utterances (V). The top row shows /dV/ sequences as in the words "deed," "dead," "dad," and "dough." The bottom row shows /dV/ sequences as in the words "dumb," "dot," "day," and "dew." The dark bands represent the first (F1) and second (F2) formant resonances.

LOCUS EQUATIONS: A METRIC
FOR DERIVING CATEGORICAL CONSTANCY
IN STOP + VOWEL UTTERANCES

Locus equations are scatterplots formed by plotting two frequency points taken from F2 transitions: (a) the onset frequency of the F2 transition immediately following the stop release burst, in relation to (b) the offset frequency of F2 measured at the vowel midpoint. The former value is plotted along the y-axis and the latter along the x-axis. Each (x, y) coordinate is thus a quantification of the F2 transition. In this simplified parametization, all frequencies between the onset and offset are ignored. Figure 2-2 shows representative locus equation plots for an adult speaker producing initial /bdg/ stops followed by 10 vowel contexts (/i, I, e, E, Q, a, o, ´, ç, u/). When such a scatterplot is generated for a given stop consonant, produced across numerous repetitions of many vowel contexts, a "normalization" of the variable F2 transitions emerges for the first time. The (x, y) coordinates for a given stop place category self-organize into a highly linear distribution across F2-defined acoustic space. These acoustically defined stop place categories, derived from only two sampling points of the dynamically changing F2 transition, can now be seen as lawful clusters of data points that are easily fit with linear regression functions.

Locus equation plots reveal that an acoustically based commonality (or constancy) actually exists within the stop place category. The commonality is not to be found in individual tokens, but rather emerges only when allophones of a stop place category are all plotted together. Another way to describe the empirical phenomenon of locus equations is to say that the inherent variability of the F2 transitions "dissolves" in the scatterplot. The normalization process happens by itself, because no complex algorithm transformed the raw frequency data.

For descriptive purposes, this tightly clustered and highly correlated distribution of F2 coordinates can be characterized by a slope and y-intercept that, importantly, varies as a direct function of place of articulation: at the lips for /b/, at the alveolar ridge for /d/, and along the hard palate for /g/. The greater the vowel's influence on the production of the stop, the steeper the slope; the less the vowel's influence on the F2 onset frequency, the flatter the slope. For example, labials, cross-linguistically, have been shown to have steeper slopes than alveolars, reflecting higher extents of

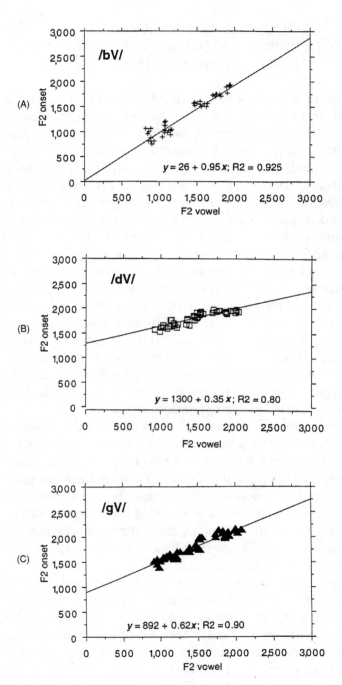

Figure 2-2. Representative locus equation scatterplots and regression functions derived from the speech of a single adult speaker. (A) Locus equation for [bV] utterances across 10 vowel contexts; (B) locus equation for [dV] utterances across 10 vowel contexts; (C) locus equation for [gV] utterances across 10 vowel contexts.

anticipatory coarticulation for labials (Sussman, Hoemeke, & Ahmed, 1993). To date, linear locus equation scatterplots have been documented for speakers of English, Swedish, Spanish, French, Arabic, Estonian, Urdu, and Thai (Sussman, Fruchter, Hilbert, & Sirosh, 1998).

The difference between the coding power of the phonological category versus individual token frequencies can be ascertained by comparing discriminant analyses using (a) token-level F2 onset/F2 vowel frequencies and (b) higher-order slope/y-intercept parameters (derived from categorical level analyses) as predictor variables. Sussman, McCaffrey, and Matthews (1991) showed that using F2 onset/offset frequencies as predictor variables accounted for 78% accuracy in classification of /bV/, /dV/, and /gV/ into the three stop place categories (chance assignment = 33%). Using locus equation slopes and y-intercepts as predictor variables led to 100% correct classification into stop place categories. This same result was also obtained in a locus equation study using Spanish speakers (Celdran & Villalba, 1995). Obviously, higher-order *category-level* parameters hold greater classificatory power than individual data points corresponding to a single CV utterance.

Some other interesting characteristics of locus equations are worth mentioning. Sussman, Fruchter, and Cable (1995) showed that locus equation scatterplots derived from bite block speech, in which speakers are asked to produce words with a bite block inserted between their back molars, reveal highly similar plots relative to normal speech produced by the same speakers. Thus, the linearity and contrastive slopes of locus equations do not depend on *specific* motoric gestures of the tongue and lips in articulating the stop + vowel sequence. In bite block speech, the tongue compensates for a stationary mandible and thus a completely different speech motor program is used to produce the same sound sequences.

In a longitudinal study examining a single infant, recorded from 7 to 16 months, Sussman, Duder, Dalston, and Cacciatore (1999) found that the "primordial CVs" of prelinguistic babbling failed to reveal the tight linear clustering universally seen in phonologically mature speakers. Such findings strongly suggest that the orderly appearance of linear locus equations develops over time and does not automatically occur simply when the vocal tract closes and subsequently opens.

Another constraint on the linear form of locus equations was uncovered when a population of children with developmental apraxia of speech (DAS) was examined (Sussman, Marquardt, &

Doyle, 2000). Locus equations obtained from children with DAS revealed highly irregular scatterplots, devoid of linearity and tight clustering of coordinates and lacking contrastive slope values to acoustically distinguish stop place contrasts. Thus, a neurologically normal motor control system would appear to be a prerequisite for the locus equation phenomenon to appear.

NEUROETHOLOGY IN THE SERVICE OF NEUROPHONETICS

The orderly and lawful form of locus equation data leads to an obvious question: Is the effect simply a phonetic epiphenomenon or does it suggest some as yet unknown functional significance for speech/language mechanisms? Our neuroethological approach to phonetics leads us to pursue the latter possibility. The first step in trying to uncover a functional significance for linear locus equation scatterplots is to find other sensory systems that, faced with similar problems of noninvariance or ambiguity in the input signal, successfully resolve the encoding problem. There are two neurophysiological studies that possess intriguing conceptual similarities to the noninvariance problem in human speech perception. The first describes how the barn owl resolves the inherent ambiguity of frequency and phase information in sound localization, and the second describes resolving stimulus variability in object recognition in monkey inferotemporal cortex. In both species, neural encoding systems, faced with processing highly variable input stimuli, achieve constancy and resolve ambiguities by using neural columns operating as the basic functional unit. This concept is referred to as "columnar absorption of variability." It is hypothesized that this neural unit is also operating in human sound processing, particularly in instances in which constancy needs to be derived from variability.

RESOLVING PHASE AMBIGUITIES IN SOUND LOCALIZATION IN THE BARN OWL

Two-eared creatures localize sound by using the time of arrival differences detected at the two ears. Jeffress (1948) had long ago conceptualized a "delay line" scenario that established a neural place code for signaling time differences of arrival between ears. Sullivan and Konishi (1986) have since verified Jeffress's notion anatomically and physiologically. Delay lines are found in the nucleus laminaris of the barn owl. They are tonotopically arranged and function as binaural phase difference detectors. Axonal signal paths from the two ears arrive at delay lines from ipsilateral and contralateral sites. The neurons forming the delay lines function as AND gates, with maximal discharge emanating from the neuron receiving simultaneous arrival of inputs from the two ears. The spatial position of the maximally active neuron in the delay line is the code for signaling on-line phase disparities, due to the longer time periods needed for axonal transmission from the lagging ear relative to the lead ear. When higher frequencies (> 1500 Hz) are present in the signal, the wavelengths of the sound are smaller than the owl's head; hence, phase differences per se become ambiguous in coding time, independently from frequency. This situation can be illustrated by considering the following example. Say a complex sound source is located 30 degrees to the right of midline. This directional source corresponds to the sound arriving at the closer right ear 50 μsec earlier than the more distant left ear. In a 2000-Hz component of the complex sound, with a period of 500 μsec, a 50-μsec time of arrival differential corresponds to a 10% phase difference between the two ears (50/500); at 3000 Hz, the same 50-μsec time differential is a 15% phase difference (50/333); at 4000 Hz, the interaural phase difference is 20% (50/250); at 5000 Hz, the phase difference is 25% (50/200); at 6000 Hz, it is 30% (50/167); at 7000 Hz, it is 35% (50/143); at 8000 Hz, it is 40% (50/125); at 9000 Hz, it is 45% (50/111); and at 10,000 Hz, it is 50% (50/100). The crucial question then becomes how the barn owl resolves this phase ambiguity inherent in the input signal.

An elegant resolution of this coding dilemma was uncovered in a study by Wagner, Takahashi, and Konishi (1987). Projections from delay line "coincidence detectors" ascend to the central nucleus of the inferior colliculus. Wagner and colleagues recorded from neurons in this nucleus that were combinatorily sensitive to various frequency/phase pairings. Their single-cell recordings showed a systematic two-dimensional mapping of frequency and phase in this nucleus (Figure 2-3). It can be seen that many of the same phase differences (plotted as a percent of a cycle) exist across the frequency axis that code a different interaural time difference (ITD). For example, a 30% phase difference at 3000 Hz signals a

100-μsec right ear lead, and the same 30% phase difference at 6000 Hz signals only a 50-μsec right ear lead. How does the barn owl know which ITD encodes accurate information for sound localization? The answer emerged when the investigators explored axonal projections to the next hierarchical processing station, the external nucleus. Neurons in this nucleus were known to be "space-specific," that is, they coded location regardless of differences in frequency or phase. Somehow, space specificity was achieved between projections from the central-to-external nuclei. When radioactive tracer substances were injected into a specific popula-

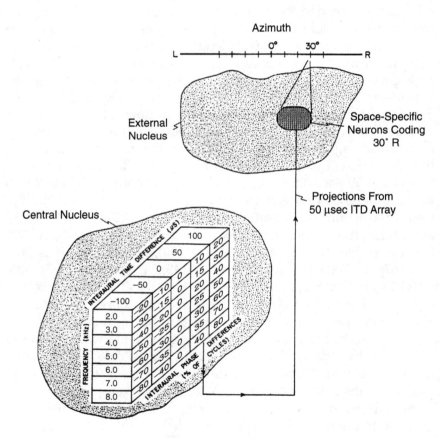

Figure 2-3. Schematic diagram. Diagram of interaural time difference (ITD) columns in the central nucleus of inferior colliculus of the barn owl and their projection to space-specific target neurons in the external nucleus mapping sound source azimuth. (From H. Sussman, "Neural coding of relational invariance in speech: Human language analogs to the barn owl," *Psychological Review, 96,* 633. Copyright 1989, American Psychological Association, Inc.)

tion of external nucleus neurons coding a particular location in space, say 30 degrees to the right, retrograde projections of the radioactive tracer showed highest concentrations in one column of the ITD arrays in the central nucleus, the column coding 50-μsec ITD (which corresponds to the specific 30-degree azimuthal location). The collective firing responses from this columnar array, *spanning all the frequency laminae*, were the ultimate source of the resolution of the phase ambiguity problem. The maximally activated column encodes the needed constancy across the variable input sensitivities to frequency and phase. What the various frequency/phase combinations share, within a given column, is that they all code the same ITD. The functional neural unit in this processing is not the single cell, but rather the collective neurons forming the ITD columns that operate as a single functional entity. The lawful variants of each column form an equivalence class coding horizontal location of an input sound. If you think of "lawful variants" as being analogous to allophones in phonetics/phonology, the link to human speech is clear.

In sound localization, the input frequencies are cotemporal in that they all are present within the complex sound arriving at the owl's ears. Locus equations present a somewhat more complicated scenario in that a speaker only hears one input sound at a time, not the whole set of allophonic variants comprising a phonological category. So the next challenge was to find a neuroethology example that more closely resembled language learning, where establishing categorical entities forming equivalence classes develop over time and with experience. Such an example can be seen in the work of Tanaka investigating visual object recognition in the macaque.

ABSORPTION OF VARIABILITY COLUMNS FOR OBJECT RECOGNITION IN THE MACAQUE

Tanaka and colleagues (Tanaka, 1993; Fujita, Tanaka, Ito, & Cheng, 1992; Tanaka, Saito, Fukada, & Moriya, 1991) recorded from single neurons in anterior inferotemporal cortex of the macaque, an area known as TE. This area is integral to processing in the ventral "what is it?" pathway of object recognition (Mishkin, Ungerleider, & Macko, 1983). Their primary goal was to uncover the selectivity properties of area TE neurons during visual object recognition. When they found a neuron that was maximally sensitive to a complex visual object, they simplified the shape, one step at a time, and systematically arrived at the most basic and essential visual features that could adequately trigger discharges from that neuron. They gradually arrived at a set of critical visual features that could, by themselves, elicit responses from single neurons in this area. When the investigators made vertical penetrations in area TE, they encountered additional neurons that shared similar or closely related visual features with the original neuron examined from that column (that was used to derive the critical features). Figure 2-4 shows a schematic diagram taken from Tanaka (1993) illustrating the "absorption of variability" columns for object recognition. In the words of Tanaka, the column "works as a buffer to absorb the changes" (p. 686). In brief, the cortical columns of area TE function collectively to create "tolerance bandwidths" for variations of visual objects. This tolerance to stimulus variability ensures a constancy of shape across the variations of the projected image on the retina. Tanaka's words best capture the essence of these columns: "This recognition is not template matching between the input image and stored images but is a flexible process in which considerable changes in images, resulting from different illumination, viewing angle, and articulation of the object, can be tolerated" (p. 685).

Because the various "visual allophones" of stimulus objects contained within a vertical column are not all present at the same

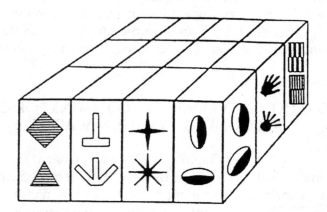

Figure 2-4. Schematic representation of columns. Columns in area TE of macaque that map lawful variants of stimulus objects. (Reprinted with permission from K. Tanaka, "Neuronal Mechanisms of Object Recognition," *Science, 262,* 686, Fig. 3. Copyright 1993 American Association for Advancement of Science.)

time, area TE columns must develop with sensory experience over time. This process more closely resembles the developmental process of a child challenged by hearing various sound combinations that he or she must organize into phonological equivalence classes possessing constancy and hence invariant phonemic structure at some level of analysis.

REPRESENTATION OF STOP + VOWEL UTTERANCES

Fine-grained distinctions among allophones fade in going from a phonetic to a phonological category (Phillips et al., 2001). This loss of fine-grained distinctions is very evident in the transform from spectrographic representations of individual stop + vowel utterances to category-level locus equation scatterplots. Specifically, individual and variable F2 transitions become irrelevant in a locus equation scatterplot. At the higher level of abstraction of the phonological category, all the parametized coordinates of F2 onsets and offsets lie together in acoustic space in a tightly clustered linear arrangement. In this context, it is intriguing that category-level quantifications of F2 onsets relative to their offsets in the vowel provide an array of data points perfectly suited to the concept of "columnar absorption of variability. " Locus equation plots for each stop place category capture the constancy that is needed to establish a viable equivalence class. All allophonic members of this category are lawfully related but highly variable, just like the variants of the critical features of Tanaka's columns in inferotemporal cortex.

In phonetic terms, the constancy coded by locus equation scatterplots is characterized by a specific slope/y-intercept. This parameter systematically varies as a function of stop place (Sussman et al., 1991). In neural-based terms, regression slopes/y-intercepts can now be reinterpreted as the collective "contents" of the neural columns. The proposal here is that neural columns, encoding F2 onset in relation to F2 vowel, can be the neural substrates suitable for mapping contrastive stop place phonological categories. All neurons within a column (or set of columns) share a sensitivity to frequency combinations having unique spatial distributions in F2-defined acoustic space. Tolerance limits exist for these combinatorial sensitivities to account for natural speaker variations. A schematic rendition of this hypothesis is shown in Figure 2-5 for /bV/, /dV/, and /gV/ utterances.

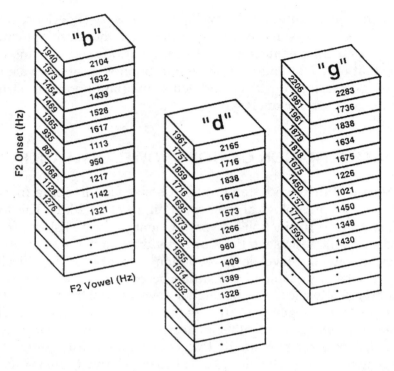

Figure 2-5. Hypothetical auditory columns encoding phonological categories for stop place. Two-dimensional arrays represent F2 onset and F2 vowel frequencies characterizing variable F2 transitions of individual speech tokens. (From H. Sussman, "Representation of Phonological Categories: A Functional Role for Auditory Columns," *Brain and Language, 80,* p. 9. Copyright 2002 Academic Press.)

Such a view is obviously based on the premise that there is an explicit isomorphism existing across acoustic-to-auditory-to-neural space. Locus equations only portray acoustic space, but it is reasonable to suppose that the brain, adept at mapping stimulus inputs possessing high degrees of statistical regularity, can readily encode such information. The precise localization of such hypothetical columns is not important at this point. In fact, there is no reason why they cannot exist at lower levels of auditory analysis corresponding to the inferior colliculus or even medial geniculate. In addition, just as the barn owl's sound localization networks process ITDs and interaural level differences in intensity in parallel for both azimuthal and elevation coordinates of the auditory map, multiple speech cues are also processed in parallel and possess extensive redundancy. In speech perception, it is well known that cues from the stop release burst (Stevens & Blumstein, 1978) and F3 onsets (Sussman, 1991) are also effective cues to signal stop place of articulation. Analogous to the barn owl example, it is highly conceivable that parallel networks processing these different aspects of the CV signal combine at higher levels of analysis to produce a more integrated representational signal.

THE IMPORTANCE OF LINEARITY

Another related aspect of locus equation data that lends itself to comparisons with neuroethology data is their extreme linear form. This current research program is investigating the precise articulatory source of this linearity. In both species examined, the avian barn owl and the mammalian bat, however, the paired acoustic components that possessed "information bearing parameters" also possessed extreme linearity (see Sussman et al., 1998). The laws of physics render phase-frequency pairings linear in the case of the barn owl, and Doppler-shifted harmonic relationships in pulse-echo biosonar processing are also strictly linear (Suga, O'Neill, Kujirai, & Manabe, 1983). What is so special about linear relationships between two input signals coding information important to a species? Learnability theory and connectionist modeling are all based on inputs possessing statistical regularities. Because higher-level auditory processing algorithms seem to be based on the operation of combination-sensitive neurons (Suga et al., 1983), it makes evolutionary sense that orderly inputs, such as highly correlated linear relationships, would make the neural encoding job easier. Perhaps elements of the complex speech signal that are maximally useful for extraction of high-information cues are the ones that possess lawful relationships. Just as the laws of physics govern the acoustic cues in neuroethology investigations, the laws of physics govern the resonance properties of the human vocal tract in forming the spectral properties of dynamically changing speech sounds.

REFERENCES

Campbell, C. B. G. (1988). In L. N. Irwin (Ed.), *Comparative neuroscience and neurobiology: Readings from the encyclopedia of neuroscience* (pp. 44–45). Boston: Birkhauser.

Celdran, E. M., & Villalba, X. (1995). Locus equations as a metric for place of articulation in automatic speech recognition. *Proceedings of the XIIIth International Congress of Phonetic Sciences (Sweden), 1,* 30–33.

Fujita, I. K., Tanaka, K., Ito, M., & Cheng, K. (1992). Columns for visual features of objects in monkey inferotemporal cortex. *Nature, 360,* 343–346.

Hauser, M. D. (1996). *The evolution of communication.* Cambridge, MA: MIT Press.

Hodos, W. (1988). Homoplasy. In L. N. Irwin (Ed.), *Comparative neuroscience and neurobiology: Readings from the encyclopedia of neuroscience* (p. 47). Boston: Birkhauser.

Jeffress, L. A. (1948). A place theory of sound localization. *Journal of Comparative and Physiological Psychology, 41,* 35–39.

Liberman, A. M., Delattre, P. C., Cooper, F. S., & Gerstman, L. J. (1954). The role of consonant-vowel transitions in the perception of the stop and nasal consonants. *Psychological Monographs, 68,* 1–13.

Mishkin, M., Ungerleider, L. G., & Macko, K. A. (1983). Object vision and spatial vision: Two central pathways. *Trends in Neuroscience, 6,* 414–417.

Phillips, C., Pellathy, T., Marantz, A., Yellin, E., Wexler, K., Poeppel, D., McGinnis, M., & Roberts, T. (2001). Auditory cortex accesses phonological categories: An MEG mismatch study. *Journal of Cognitive Neuroscience, 12*(6), 1038–1055.

Stevens, K. N., & Blumstein, S. (1978). Invariant cues for place of articulation in stop consonants. *Journal of the Acoustical Society of America, 64,* 1358–1368.

Suga, N., O'Neill, W. E., Kujirai, K., & Manabe, T. (1983). Specificity of combination-sensitive neurons for processing of complex biosonar signals in auditory cortex of the mustached bat. *Neurophysiology, 49,* 1573–1627.

Sullivan, W. E., & Konishi, M. (1986). Neural map of interaural phase differences in the owl's brainstem. *Proceedings of the National Academy of Sciences (USA), 83,* 8400–8404.

Sussman, H. M. (1991). The representation of stop consonants in three-dimensional acoustic space. *Phonetica, 48,* 18–31.

Sussman, H. M., Duder, C., Dalston, E., & Cacciatore, A. (1999). An acoustic analysis of the development of CV coarticulation: A case study. *Journal of Speech, Language, and Hearing Research, 42,* 1080–1096.

Sussman, H. M., Fruchter, D., & Cable, A. (1995). Locus equations derived from compensatory articulation. *Journal of the Acoustical Society of America, 97*, 3112–3124.

Sussman, H. M., Fruchter, D., Hilbert, J., & Sirosh, J. (1998). Linear correlates in the speech signal: The orderly output constraint. *Behavioral and Brain Sciences, 21*(2), 241–299.

Sussman, H. M., Hoemeke, K., & Ahmed, F. (1993). A cross-linguistic investigation of locus equations as a relationally invariant descriptor for place of articulation. *Journal of the Acoustical Society of America, 94*, 1256–1268.

Sussman, H. M., Marquardt, T. P., & Doyle, J. (2000). An acoustic analysis of phonemic integrity and contrastiveness in developmental apraxia of speech. *Journal of Medical Speech-Language Pathology, 8*, 301–313.

Sussman, H. M., McCaffrey, H. A., & Matthews, S. A. (1991). An investigation of locus equations as a source of relational invariance for stop place categorization. *Journal of the Acoustical Society of America, 90*, 1309–1325.

Tanaka, K. (1993). Neuronal mechanisms of object recognition. *Science, 262*, 685–688.

Tanaka, K., Saito, H., Fukada, M., & Moriya, M. (1991). Coding visual images of objects in the inferotemporal cortex of the macaque monkey. *Journal of Neurophysiology, 66*, 170–189.

Wagner, H., Takahashi, T., & Konishi, M. (1987). Representation of intraural time difference in the central nucleus of the barn owl's inferior colliculus. *Journal of Neuroscience, 7*, 3105–3116.

3

Time Series Analyses of Spike Trains: Identifying Nonlinear Deterministic Structure

Carmen C. Canavier, Ph.D.
Department of Psychology
University of New Orleans
New Orleans, LA

Lee P. Lovejoy
M.D./Ph.D. Program
University of California at San Diego
San Diego, CA

Siva R. Perla
Department of Psychology
University of New Orleans
New Orleans, LA

Paul D. Shepard
Maryland Psychiatric Research Center
University of Maryland School of Medicine
Baltimore, MD

In the auditory system, as in the remainder of the nervous system, information is transmitted primarily by action potentials (spikes). Electrophysiological data are frequently acquired in the form of a series of spike times or, equivalently, a series of interspike intervals (ISIs). Analysis of this type of data includes ISI histograms and statistical measures such as the coefficient of variation (CV, or the standard deviation divided by the mean) and the Fano factor (the variance divided by the mean). These measures are insensitive to the precise order in which the interspike intervals occur. This order is unimportant if information is transmitted using a frequency code, in which spike frequency is averaged across a population of neurons over a short time interval or, alternatively, across a single neuron over a longer time interval. The precise ordering of ISIs, however, may be important in terms of signal processing if a temporal coding scheme rather than a frequency code is employed. In addition, and more directly relevant to the subject matter of this chapter, the precise ordering of ISIs may be useful in determining the underlying mechanisms responsible for the variability in interspike intervals. This chapter introduces a method of identifying certain types of nonlinear deterministic structure in spike trains and then suggests how this method might be applied to auditory spike trains.

ISIs MAY BE PREDICTABLE

The variabilities exhibited by series of ISIs recorded in the cochlear and vestibular components of the eighth cranial vestibulocochlear nerve serve as examples of two qualitatively and statistically distinct types of variability. Trains of action potentials recorded from the vestibular nerve appear to fit the traditional statistical model of a population of integrate and fire neurons: events that lead to a suprathreshold depolarization appear to occur with an approximately exponential distribution about a mean, resulting in a distribution of interevent times that is nearly identical to that of a stochastic Poisson process. The caveat that the distribution is nearly exponential results from neural biophysics that dictate the existence of an absolute and a relative refractory period, so that very short ISIs are nonphysiological and cannot be observed. In contrast, trains of action potentials recorded from the cochlear nerve do not fit such a model. A Poisson point process is by definition memoryless: each interval is completely independent of all previous intervals, and a Fano factor plot for such a process is flat. For actual data from the auditory nerve, when sufficiently long time windows are examined (0.1–100 sec), the Fano factor appears to increase as a power law function of time for trains of action potentials recorded spontaneously or in response to a pure tone (Teich, 1992), implying a memory mechanism. In an attempt to include a memory mechanism in their stochastic model of auditory nerve firing, Lowen and Teich (1991) showed that such statistics could be reproduced by two Poisson generators, with the output of the first becoming the input to a linear filter with a power law impulse response function. The output of the linear filter is a memory mechanism that provides a variable mean for the second Poisson generator. The output of this stochastic model is a fractal point process.

The above-mentioned stochastic models and statistical methods do not attempt to exploit any clues regarding the nature of the memory mechanism provided by the exact ordering of the ISIs. Physiological neurons have access to numerous biophysical and biochemical parameters that could serve as substrates for the memory mechanisms that create dependence of the ISI on previous ISIs. Teich and Lowen (1994) have suggested that calcium levels in the hair cell or levels of neurotransmitter in the hair cell to auditory neuron synapse could provide a memory of the type that they implemented as the variable mean of the second stochastic process. Dynamic models that represent neurons in terms of the activation (and inactivation) states of their ion channel populations, membrane potential, and certain intracellular ionic concentrations can capture essential aspects of the nonlinear dynamics of the excitable neuron. Deterministic models with only a few such variables can produce trains of action potentials that appear stochastic but are in fact deterministic and chaotic, in either a spontaneous or a driven mode (Glass & Mackey, 1988). An excitable cell can always be biased into a periodic oscillatory regime, in which the values of the state variable change in tandem, tracing out a limit cycle (see Figure 3-1, part A2) in the space whose coordinates do not include time, but only the state variables themselves. The position along this limit cycle is the phase of the system, and small perturbations (synaptic noise) would tend to preferentially perturb the phase rather than the amplitude of the oscillation (Oprisan & Canavier, 2002). Therefore, synaptic noise cannot be treated as additive noise, but rather as multiplicative noise. A chaotic oscillation also traces a characteristic path in the state space (see Figure 3-1, part B2), but this path follows a chaotic attractor that is geometrically fractal, rather than a simple closed curve that constitutes a limit cycle. Position in the state space relative to the appropriate attractor is clearly a memory mechanism. In fact, memory mechanisms at differing time scales are possible because

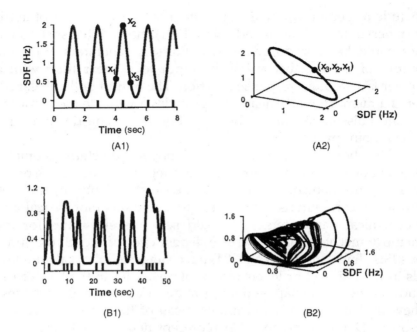

Figure 3-1. Reconstruction of an attractor from a spike density function (SDF). (A1) SDF of periodic spike train generated by a model neuron. Spikes are shown as a comb plot on the x-axis. An example of three time-delayed coordinates corresponding to a single point on the attractor is indicated as x_1, x_2, and x_3. (A2) The reconstructed limit cycle attractor. (B1) SDF of chaotic spike train generated by a model neuron. (B2) The reconstructed chaotic attractor. (Adapted from L. P. Lovejoy, P. D. Shepard, and C. C. Canavier, Apamin-induced irregular firing *in vitro* and irregular firing observed *in vivo* in dopamine neurons is chaotic, *Neuroscience, 104,* 829–840. Copyright 2001. With permission from Elsevier Science.)

the speed of relaxation back to the attractor depends on absolute position in the space as well as on the direction of motion.

The structure of the attractor provides not only a mechanism for memory, but also a mechanism for predicting future activity based on this memory. In the case of a limit cycle, once the attractor is known and a position on it is specified, the future trajectory of the oscillator in the absence of any noise can be predicted for all time with perfect accuracy. Of course, every physical system is noisy. Additive noise degrades the accuracy of predictions of future trajectories, but the degradation is not cumulative. Prediction of a periodic oscillation at any time in the future should have roughly a fixed amount error in the presence of a constant level of uncorrelated additive noise (Sugihara & May, 1990). On the other hand, the degradation of accuracy produced by the multiplicative noise introduced by synaptic noise is cumulative, causing predictions a short time into the future to be more accurate than those a longer time into the future (Lovejoy, Shepard, & Canavier, 2001).

A train of action potentials with ISIs distributed as the interevent times in a stochastic Poisson process has no deterministic attractor structure that can be exploited and cannot be predicted using the technique described above, or any other technique, because the process is by definition memoryless. Certain types of correlated noise do have structure that could be exploited for predictive purposes, but this structure is not deterministic. The accuracy of a prediction, or forecast, can be quantified by using the Pearson's correlation coefficient (r) between the actual time series and the forecast. The error can then be quantified as $(1 - r)$. For certain types of correlated noise, the degradation of the prediction with increasing forecast horizon can be quantified. A trajectory produced by a fractal Brownian motion has no deterministic structure. Yet nonlinear prediction techniques are more accurate at predicting short intervals into the future than long, because the current position of a trajectory provides some clues as to the future position of the trajectory that a nonlinear prediction algorithm can exploit. The error $(1 - r)$ is a power law curve of prediction time (Tsonis & Elsner, 1992) with the slope of a log-log plot determined by the reciprocal of the fractal dimension, which also controls the variance as a function of time. On the other hand, for a deterministic chaotic time series, the error is an exponential function of prediction time, with the slope on a semilog plot related to the positive Lyaponov exponent on the attractor (Wales, 1991).

FORECASTING USING RECONSTRUCTED ATTRACTORS

If the deterministic dynamic mechanisms described above are responsible for the timing of action potentials, it should be possible to reconstruct the attractor from a time series (Packard, Crutchfield, Farmer, & Shaw, 1980) of the action potentials. The spike train data, however, do not contain an evenly sampled time series of the membrane potential or any other state variable but rather a record of the times at which the membrane potential exceeds a certain threshold, so a great deal of information regarding the dynamic system is unavailable. Under some circumstances, the ISIs can be used directly to forecast future ISIs accurately (Racicot & Longtin, 1997; Sauer, 1994), but the independent variable is not time, but rather spike number. Thus, all temporal scaling is lost, so that nonlinear prediction can identify nonlinear structure, but the distinct scaling characteristics of chaotic activity cannot be identified. In addition, the temporal resolution is on the order of a trip around the attractor. The exponential scaling characteristic of chaos results from divergence of trajectories on the attractor and is only evident at relatively short time scales because once the trajectories diverge to opposite ends of the attractor, they can diverge no farther. Thus, the first need is to construct a time series from the ISI data. One method of constructing a continuous function of time from a spike train is the spike density function (SDF) (Szucs, 1998). SDFs were constructed by convolving a window function, such as a Gaussian, with a pulse train created by putting a pulse at each recorded spike time (see Figure 3-1, parts A1 and B1).

To reconstruct an attractor in state space, multiple variables are required. A common method of recovering the geometry of an attractor from a time series of a single variable is to use time-delayed samples of the single variable as additional variables (Packard et al., 1980) so that each point is associated with a vector (x_1, x_2, x_3), where $x_1 = x(t)$, $x_2 = x(t + \tau)$, $x_3 = x(t + 2\tau)$, and τ is a time lag. Each point can then be plotted in the appropriate state space. The selection of the number of points in the vector and the time lag $\tau\tau$ between them is not trivial and will not be covered here. The procedure is illustrated in Figure 3-1 using a neural model (Plant & Kim, 1976) biased either in a periodic oscillatory regime (Figure 3-1, parts A1 and A2) or a known chaotic regime (Figure 3-1, parts B1 and B2) (see Canavier, Clark, & Byrne, 1990). The SDF generated by the model neuron was divided into two parts. The first part was used to reconstruct the time series as shown in Figure 3-1, parts A1 and B1. Then a prediction was made by associating each point in the second part with the appropriate vector, determining the points on the attractor that bracketed the vector, and using the known future trajectories of the points on the attractor to estimate the future trajectory of the point in the second part of the data for a given forecast horizon (prediction time) into the future. This procedure produced a predicted SDF at each prediction interval as shown in Figure 3-2 using the simulated chaotic attractor as

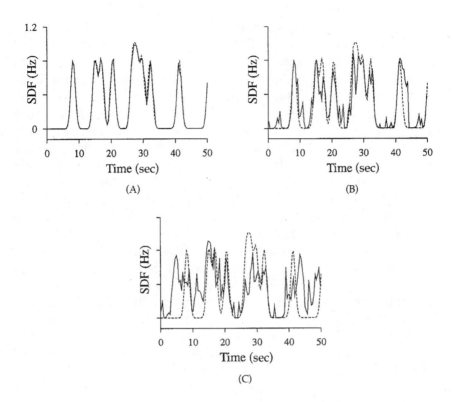

Figure 3-2. Comparison of predicted and actual SDF for simulated chaotic regime. The time step into the future is indicated by p and the correlation coefficient by r. The actual SDF is shown using a dotted line in all cases and the prediction using a solid line. The x-axis indicates actual time within the SDF, as contrasted with prediction time steps p given in the caption. (A) $p = 1$, $r = 0.99$. (B) $p = 5$, $r = 0.84$. (C) $p = 10$, $r = 0.46$. (Adapted from L. P. Lovejoy, P. D. Shepard, and C. C. Canavier, Apamin-induced irregular firing *in vitro* and irregular firing observed *in vivo* in dopamine neurons is chaotic, *Neuroscience, 104,* 829–840. Copyright 2001. With permission from Elsevier Science.)

an example. The actual second part of the time series is also shown at each prediction step (1, 5, and 10 time steps). A time step equal to one tenth the average ISI was used.

The nonlinear prediction method forecast the simulated pacemaker (another name for a regular, limit cycle oscillator) perfectly, which is not surprising in view of its periodic nature. What is more surprising is that an excellent prediction was obtained of the SDF resulting from the action potential train generated by the Plant and Kim model in a known chaotic regime, and that predictability appeared to fall off exponentially. Clearly, the reconstructed "attractors" do not capture all aspects of the model that produced the action potentials. The original attractor of the Plant and Kim model comprises six state variables, has a very asymmetric amplitude distribution about its mean, and is time irreversible. Although this study did not try to forecast time-reversed or amplitude inverted versions of the SDF, it is not likely that such forecasts would differ significantly for the periodic SDF, indicating that the forecast method only detects linear structure (Stam, Pijn, & Pritchard, 1998) in the case of the reconstructed pacemaker. Although the "attractor" reconstructed in the chaotic case does look chaotic because it seemingly possesses a self-similar structure and although the forecast appears to scale exponentially, the predictive ability falls off much more rapidly than that of a forecast performed directly on the slowest variable of the original dynamical model. Shuffling the intervals (not shown), however, destroys the exponential decay and degrades the predictability, indicating that in the chaotic case, temporal structure is indeed detected and exploited by the nonlinear prediction method.

The parameters of the Gaussian window were chosen so that the pulse train was converted into a continuous function with a sharp peak in its Fourier transform at the spiking frequency. One problem with applying nonlinear prediction to the SDF is that the Gaussian window itself imparts spurious predictability to the SDF. This spurious predictability was examined by applying the nonlinear prediction algorithm to an SDF generated from a spike train whose interspike intervals were generated by a simulated Poisson process. The intervals themselves were inherently unpredictable, but the SDF exhibited a predictability that scaled more rapidly than exponentially (Figure 3-3, part A, triangles). We are investigating solving this problem using a window function whose shape depends on the ISI, because although we could avoid being fooled by the spurious predictability in the case of the model data, in the case of the experimental data (Figure 3-3, part B), we have not yet been able to distinguish between the predictability of the original spike train and its shuffled surrogates.

Another test of the method was to see how the predictability of a nonlinear periodic oscillator degraded in the presence of simulated synaptic noise. The synaptic noise was simulated by assuming that the interevent times between synaptic inputs were distributed as those of a Poisson process. The perturbation in synaptic conductance was simulated as the response of a damped second-order

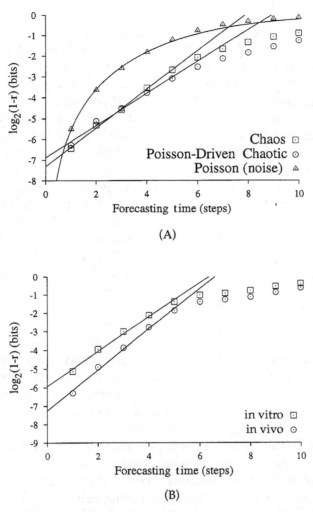

Figure 3-3. Summary of exponential scaling obtained for noisy, noisy chaotic, chaotic, and putative chaotic spike density functions. The plots shown are semilog so that an exponential relationship (and only such a relationship) will appear as a straight line. (A) Spurious predictability of a spike train whose ISIs are distributed as the interevent times of a Poisson process (triangles) resulting in faster than exponential increase in error, exponential increase in error resulting from a spike train generated by simulated chaotic dynamics (squares), and a similar exponential increase in error for the same chaotic dynamics in the presence of simulated synaptic noise (circles). (B) Exponential increase in prediction error with forecast time for experimentally recorded ISIs for the spontaneous in vivo case (circles) and data recorded in a slice in the presence of apamin (squares). (Adapted from L. P. Lovejoy, P. D. Shepard, and C. C. Canavier, Apamin-induced irregular firing *in vitro* and irregular firing observed *in vivo* in dopamine neurons is chaotic, *Neuroscience, 104*, 829–840. Copyright 2001. With permission from Elsevier Science.)

linear oscillator to a square pulse (Canavier, Clark, Baxter, & Byrne, 1993). Although the perturbations did not perceptibly change the appearance of the SDF (not shown), they caused the reconstructed attractor to spread out in the state space (see Figure 3-4, part A1). For simplicity, each perturbation was identical, and they were excitatory postsynaptic potentials. The Plant and Kim oscillator in the parameter regime chosen produced only phase advances in response to these perturbations, which is characteristic of Type I excitability (Oprisan & Canavier, 2002); thus, the total phase resetting increased with time (with the caveat that resetting by a full cycle is indistinguishable from no resetting). Because the average frequency is predictable but the phase resetting is random, the predictability of the time series should decay with forecast time. Because the phase resetting produced by an individual perturbation was small, the predictability decayed gradually (Figure 3-4, part A2). A similar gradual decay of predictability was produced by others using nonlinear forecasting to predict a time series generated by a stochastic linear model with a very narrow power spectrum (Stam et al., 1998), so additional tests are required to prove nonlinear structure.

The effect of synaptic noise on the simulated chaotic regime was also examined. For additive noise in a chaotic regime, a constant offset is added to the expected exponential decay. Little effect was found on the exponential increase in error in the prediction of the chaotic SDF with and without small amounts of synaptic noise as described above (Figure 3-3, part A).

The next step was to apply the nonlinear forecasting techniques to SDF generated by experimentally observed ISI data from mammalian midbrain neurons. These data were of interest because it was suspected that a pharmaceutical agent, apamin, was capable of converting a noisy limit cycle oscillator into a chaotic oscillator. The dopamine neurons of the substantia nigra pars compacta fire action potentials spontaneously, and in a regular pacemaker-like fashion when they are isolated from many of their synaptic afferents in a slice preparation. In contrast, these same neurons frequently fire irregularly when the recordings are obtained in an in vivo setting. Interestingly, the application of apamin to a slice preparation induces irregular firing that is qualitatively similar to the irregular firing observed in vivo (Ping & Shepard, 1996; Shepard & Bunney, 1988). Application of the delay embedding attractor reconstruction and nonlinear forecasting techniques to the experimentally generated SDFs produced results similar to those obtained for certain simulated cases. The regular

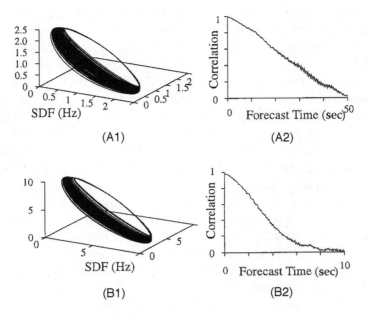

Figure 3-4. Comparison of simulated and experimental noisy limit cycles. (A1) Simulated limit cycle oscillator with synaptic noise. (A2) Decay of prediction accuracy as measured by the correlation coefficient with forecast time. Approximately 35 cycles are contained in a 50-sec forecast interval. (B1) Attractor reconstruction from experimental data for regular firing of dopamine neurons in a slice preparation. (B2) Approximately 30 cycles are contained in the 10-sec forecast interval. (Adapted from L. P. Lovejoy, P. D. Shepard, and C. C. Canavier, Apamin-induced irregular firing *in vitro* and irregular firing observed *in vivo* in dopamine neurons is chaotic, *Neuroscience, 104,* 829–840. Copyright 2001. With permission from Elsevier Science.)

firing in the slice preparation resembled the limit cycle oscillation with synaptic noise both in the "spread out" appearance of the attractor (Figure 3-4, part B1) and in the gradual decrease in predictability (Figure 3-4, part B2). The irregular firing observed both in the presence of apamin in the slice preparation and spontaneously in the in vivo recordings had prediction errors that increased exponentially (Figure 3-3B), but as mentioned above, the problem of spurious predictability has not yet been resolved.

There is a significant difference between midbrain dopamine neurons and auditory neurons with respect to the application of nonlinear forecasting methods to detect nonlinear deterministic structure. Whereas dopamine neurons are known to fire regularly and spontaneously in a slice preparation, justifying the assumption that they can be characterized as limit cycle oscillators in certain parametric regimes, spontaneous regular firing has not been observed to our knowledge in auditory neurons. Data from auditory neurons, however, are frequently obtained under conditions of periodic forcing, such as recordings of auditory nerve fiber in the presence of a pure tone stimulus. Under these conditions, irregular firing can result from the interaction of the intrinsic nonlinear dynamics of a neuron and the periodic forcing. Spikes recorded in response to a pure tone tend to occur near a particular phase of the stimulus, but may skip one or more cycles between firing, hence the large irregularity. This irregularity may be stochastic—a result of a random walk in membrane potential near the threshold, for example—or it may result from deterministic chaos. Unfortunately, such chaos might be impossible to detect from the threshold crossings (spike times) alone, because subthreshold activity (Kaplan et al., 1996) may cause interspike intervals of similar length to be qualitatively different in the number of subthreshold responses they contain. Nonlinear forecasting performed directly on the ISIs failed to provide evidence for a deterministic rather than a random origin for the variability in auditory neuron ISIs (Longtin, 1993), but a dependence on stimulus phase was observed. An approach using an attractor reconstructed from SDFs, with stimulus phase incorporated into the analysis, might be more sensitive to the detection of deterministic chaos, if it is present in the system. The suspicion is that both stochastic and deterministic mechanisms contribute to spike train variability.

ACKNOWLEDGMENTS

This work was funded by NIH grants NS37963 (CCC) and MH48543 (PDS).

REFERENCES

Canavier, C. C., Clark, J. W., Baxter, D. A., & Byrne, J. H. (1993). Nonlinear dynamics in a model neuron provide a novel mechanisms for transient synaptic inputs to produce long-term alterations of postsynaptic activity. *Journal of Neurophysiology, 69,* 2252–2257.

Canavier, C. C., Clark, J. W., & Byrne, J. H. (1990). Routes to chaos in a model of a bursting neuron. *Biophysical Journal, 57,* 1245–1251.

Glass, L., & Mackey, M. C. (1988). From clocks to chaos: The rhythms of life. Princeton, NJ: Princeton University Press.

Kaplan, D. T., Clay, J. R., Manning, T., Glass, L., Guevara, M. R., & Shrier, A. (1996). Subthreshold dynamics of periodically stimulated squid giant axons. *Physical Review Letters, 76,* 4074–4077.

Longtin, A. (1993). Nonlinear forecasting of spike trains from sensory neurons. *International Journal of Chaos and Bifurcations, 3,* 651–661.

Lovejoy, L. P., Shepard, P. D., & Canavier, C. C. (2001). Apamin-induced irregular firing *in vitro* and irregular firing observed *in vivo* in dopamine neurons is chaotic. *Neuroscience, 104,* 829–840.

Lowen, S. B., & Teich, M. C. (1991). Doubly stochastic Poisson point process driven by fractal shot noise. *Physical Review Letters A, 43,* 4192–4215.

Oprisan, S. A., & Canavier, C. C. (2002). The influence of the limit cycle topology on phase resetting curve. *Neural Computation, 14,* 1027–1057.

Packard, N. H., Crutchfield, J. P., Farmer, J. D., & Shaw, R. S. (1980). Geometry from a time series. *Physical Review Letters, 45,* 712–716.

Ping, H. X., & Shepard, P. D. (1996). Apamin-sensitive Ca^{2+}-activated K^+ channels regulate pacemaker activity in nigral dopamine neurons. *NeuroReport, 7,* 809–814.

Plant, R. E., & Kim, M. (1976). Mathematical description of a bursting pacemaker neuron by a modification of the Hodgkin-Huxley equations. *Biophysical Journal, 16,* 227–244.

Racicot, D. M., & Longtin, A. (1997). Interspike interval attractors from chaotically driven neuron models. *Physica D, 104,* 184–204.

Sauer, T. (1994). Reconstruction of dynamical systems from interspike intervals. *Physical Review Letters, 72,* 3811–3814.

Shepard, P. D., & Bunney, B. S. (1988). Effects of apamin on the discharge properties of putative dopamine-containing neurons in vitro. *Brain Research, 463,* 380–384.

Stam, C. J., Pijn, J. P. M., & Pritchard, W. S. (1998). Reliable detection of nonlinearity in experimental time series with strong periodic components. *Physica D, 112,* 361–380.

Sugihara G., & May, R. M. (1990). Nonlinear forecasting as a way of distinguishing chaos from measurement error in time series. *Nature, 358,* 217–220.

Szucs, A. (1998). Applications of the spike density function in analysis of neuronal firing patterns. *Journal of Neuroscience Methods, 81,* 159–167.

Teich, M. C. (1992). Fractal neuronal firing patterns. In T. McKenna, J. Davis, & S. F. Zornetzer (Eds.), *Single neuron computation* (pp. 589–625). Boston: Academic.

Teich, M. C., & Lowen. S. B. (1994). Fractal patterns in auditory nerve-spike trains. *IEEE Engineering in Medicine and Biology Magazine, 13*(2), 197–202.

Tsonis, A. A., & Elsner, J. B. (1992). Nonlinear prediction as a way of distinguishing chaos from random fractal sequences. *Nature, 358,* 217–220.

Wales, D. J. (1991). Calculating the rate of loss of information from a chaotic time series by forecasting. *Nature, 370,* 485–488.

4

Understanding Neural Circuits

Theodore G. Weyand, Ph.D.
Department of Cell Biology and Anatomy
Louisiana State University Health Sciences Center
New Orleans, LA

ABSTRACT

The brain is a massively parallel and complicated analogue machine. Nonetheless, it is deterministic, and studying the activity of the neurons that make up the brain offers a promising method for understanding the brain and the mind. The neuron doctrine is an important concept that simplifies the problem of understanding the mind from a relatively vague concept to a more tractable problem of understanding the neuron. Implementation of the neuron doctrine depends, first, on the ability to describe isomorphic relations between the activity of a neuron and events in the world (the "receptive field") and, second, on explaining how these properties of the neuron emerge from the circuitry within which the neuron is embedded. The heuristics needed to characterize the isomorphic relations require some a priori knowledge of what the brain computes and draws significantly on insights from psychology and artificial intelligence. Understanding how the receptive field properties emerge from the properties of its inputs is problematic, because the brain is neither hierarchical nor strictly parallel, nor does it behaves linearly. Enough success has been achieved, however, to indicate that the neuron doctrine continues to be the most promising approach to a mechanical solution to mind.

INTRODUCTION

The human brain contains over a billion neurons. Under-standing what these neurons do and how they do it would be equivalent to understanding the mind, a formidable challenge. To the extent that it is a comfort, it is reasonable to assume that whatever processes account for mind are grounded in physics and natural law. As such, one can say that there is a mechanical solution for the mind. Of course, the solution is complex. Witness, for example, the frustrations engineers have had in building machines that see, hear, or act, activities animals with only a few hundred neurons do effortlessly. The brain is a computational device. Problems in understanding the rules of computation have more to do with the complexity of the system rather than lend support to the idea that the brain operates outside the realm of known physics. Although it is possible that the nature of brains could somehow enable them to act as a conduit to another dimension, or operate as a telemetric receiver from some as yet unnamed higher power in a galaxy far away, parsimony argues otherwise. The purpose of this chapter is to delineate from a computational and abstract view what the brain does and how it does it. Only two assumptions are made: the neuron is the fundamental unit to be understood, and action potentials ("spikes," brief and uniform pulses of electrical signals) originating in these neurons are the temporally discrete carriers of information.

It is sometimes argued that computers are not brains and that therefore the mind cannot be understood using computational solutions. Perhaps this argument emerges because the problem is taken too literally. The interest here is in the message, the processes of the mind, not the medium in which it dwells. The medium is simply the physical architecture through which the message passes. What are sought are the algorithms that bind initial conditions to final conditions. Computers can simulate any process, but the algorithms, the rules by which some transform should be achieved, must be supplied. Identifying these algorithms is the central problem of understanding the brain. Mathematics is the descriptor and is simply a collection of rules. Probable success is when the simulation matches the behavior. To argue that there is something "special" about the medium is as silly as arguing that doing calculations using a slide rule is fundamentally different from doing calculations using an electronic calculator. Yes, the tools calculate differently, and one is a little more accurate than the other, but two times two is still four on both.

WHAT DO BRAINS "DO"?

Brains are usually thought of as taking in information from the world, processing it in some way, and then initiating some action as a result of the process. This characterization is reasonable, but to understand the process better, it is instructive to consider a simpler system whose behavior is captured by the same description but that has no neurons. Consider the world of the billiard ball sitting on a pool table. It "behaves" in the sense that when a force such as that imposed on it by the cue ball or another billiard ball hits it, the resulting acceleration, velocity, and trajectory of its path can be predicted quite well. The factors that influence its behavior are a finite set, and, to a player, incident angle of the hitting object is probably most important. There are other factors that will determine the ball's behavior, such as velocity of the hitting object, friction of the surface, and stiffness of the objects, but this list is short and the equations to describe the ball's behavior are known and relatively simple. An important yet perhaps radical notion is whether to consider the billiard ball as possessing knowledge of the world. In fact, the billiard ball has attributes, and these attributes—weight, smoothness, rigidity, size—dictate its behavior, and that will pass for knowledge. Except for scale, it is not clear that a brain is any different. Concepts such as "choice" and "plasticity" are the result of complexity (scaling up) of the system, nothing more. In this example, the transparency between what the world imposes on the object and the object's behavior is relatively simple, and the direct result of the object's properties, that is, the object's knowledge of the world. This transparency can be described by applying nothing more than a small set of equations known to Newton.

THE NEURON DOCTRINE

The billiard ball, of course, is not really a brain, but one can appreciate that its behavior is constrained by its physical attributes and, under these conditions, is knowledge. The goal of neuroscience is to explain the brain as precisely as one can discuss the actions of the billiard ball. This explanation should be given in terms of a transform, in which the appropriate parameters comprising the input are described, the mathematical operations imposed, and a behavior or a class of behaviors documented as output. For the brain, the neuron is the appropriate level of description; therefore, its output—action potentials—is the appropriate level of information to be understood. Historically, this metric has been fruitful and is the basis for the *neuron doctrine* (reviewed in Barlow, 1972, 1995). The tactic is exceedingly simple: treat the brain as an input/output device, and because the brain is divided into clusters, parts, or modules, treat these entities as input/output devices as well. Knowledge of where these entities lie on a chain will allow further comment on how the transforms are done. This approach can accommodate plasticity, learning, and so forth by assuming that the device is a dynamic. For example, if the rigidity of the billiard ball were variable (i.e, it was elastic), the ball's behavior would certainly change. Rigidity, originally a fixed parameter, would now have to be assigned as a variable. As an empirical issue, the advantage of the neuron doctrine is that it greatly simplifies the problem. Mechanical solutions to mind can now be addressed as mechanical solutions to neurons. Success of the neuron doctrine turns on the ability to answer these two basic questions:

What does the neuron know about the world?
How does the neuron know about the world?

Neither question is easy to answer. The answer to the first requires some understanding of what the brain does as a computational problem. The answer to the second requires appreciation of the computational architecture of the brain.

What Does the Neuron Know About the World?

If one uses a microelectrode and records the pattern of action potentials produced by a neuron, for most neurons it becomes readily apparent that the activity is modulated either by events in the world or by the activity of the animal. The observation that neurons have selectivity for only certain events is the basis for the term *receptive field*. The receptive field identifies events, appropriately known as "trigger features, that cause the neuron to discharge spikes or action potentials. For example, one can describe visual neurons that discharge strongly (are "triggered") to a stimulus moving in one direction but not other directions of motion. In addition to trigger features, many neurons are sensitive over only a spatially restricted region of a sensory surface or only access a restricted set of the musculature. Thus, for the example of the direction selective neuron, its spatial selectivity would reference that it only responded to motion in a limited portion of the visual field.

How Does the Neuron Know About the World?

The description of the receptive field is the first step of the neuron doctrine. It tells us what the neuron knows. The second step is to explain how those properties emerged. For the example of the direction selective cell described above, Barlow and Levick (1965) provided a plausible mechanism. Movement of a stimulus through the receptive field in one direction yields a vigorous response, whereas movement of a stimulus through the receptive field in the opposite direction yields a poor response. Moving stimuli through the receptive field in other directions yields responses proportional to their proximity to the preferred vector. A key observation these investigators made was that if the stimulus were moved very slowly, the directionality of the cell disappeared. They then reasoned that the mechanism of directional selectivity emerged via some asymmetric circuits that inhibited responses to movement in one direction but not the other. The inhibition was temporal constrained, maximal at first and falling as a leaky integrator. The temporal constraint yielded an inhibition constrained by stimulus velocity. Barlow and Levick's "model" could be implemented with an array of phototransistors (electronic elements whose output varied with light levels) fed to logic circuits (transistor elements that perform logical operations such as putting out a pulse when one input or the other was asserted; commonly called OR gates). The model appears to mimic the observed properties and as such "explains" directional selectivity, because one can build such a circuit.

BARRIERS TO THE NEURON DOCTRINE

Because the neuron doctrine assigns causality of mental operations to the muttering of neurons (spikes), it is a potentially powerful method of explaining the mind because, as outlined above, it shifts understanding the mind to the much more tractable problem of understanding the receptive field properties of the single neuron. Nonetheless, barriers to the success of the neuron doctrine are formidable. In the example above, Barlow and Levick (1965) succeeded at providing a mechanism for direction selectivity for several reasons. First, the investigators were bright and observant, but they were also lucky. They had happened upon a robust and interesting property in the retina, only two or three synapses removed from the photoreceptors. The properties of neurons near sensory surfaces are usually easier to understand than other neurons, probably because they derive so much of their input from simple properties as the presence or absence of light. As one goes deeper into the brain, however, things get complicated for two reasons: the trigger features get more persnickety (a phenomenon called "sparse" coding), and the circuits within which these neurons are embedded are more complicated. These two factors place serious constraints on the success of the neuron doctrine.

Barrier 1: Characterizing the Receptive Field

The receptive field is central to the neuron doctrine; it describes what the neuron knows about the world. As a practical matter, it involves using microelectrodes to eavesdrop on individual neurons as they go about their daily chores. It is often technically challenging, but the agenda is straightforward: search for isomorphic relations between events/activities and activity of the neuron. The truly difficult problem is identifying what constitutes the trigger features. For a sensory/perceptual system, there are an infinite number of potential events (stimuli) to which one can expose the neuron. How does one find the events that capture the trigger features? A number of factors influence the investigator's decisions on which stimuli or which tasks will most likely reveal the neuron's trigger features.

Anatomy. The location of the neuron is an important clue about what sorts of events might trigger the neuron. If the neuron is in the retina (the tissue in the back of the eyeball that contains the photoreceptors), it is a good guess that the neuron has something to do with vision. Similarly, if the neuron is within a structure that receives significant input from the retina, a selectivity for some visual event is suspected. Similar logic could be applied to making sounds when recording from the neurons and fibers of the cochlea (containing the mechanoreceptors that give rise to hearing), or tapping the body when recording from the fibers that innervate the skin. This logic applies to the motor domain as well. If the anatomy indicates that the neuron is wired to a muscle, it is a good guess that the neuron's activity is directly related to the observed movement of that muscle. Related to anatomy would be stimulation experiments. For example, if one stimulates a structure that causes the animal's eyes to move, it would then be reasonable to study the activity of neurons in that structure when the animal makes eye movements.

Trauma/ablation. The changes in behavior as a result of either deliberate or accidental damage to a structure offer the investigator important clues as to what the neurons in the structure might be doing. For example, the inability to create new memories following damage to the hippocampus has led investigators to intensive study of the activity of this structure during learning tasks. Another example is the observation that patients with damage to their supplementary motor cortex fail to have adaptive motor strategies led investigators to discover neurons selective for pieces of motor acts only when they were executed in sequence (e.g., Tanji & Shima, 1994).

Psychophysics. Characterizing what the animal is capable of detecting has been a valuable source of clues. This category includes ethology, the study of animal behavior. A good knowledge of the animal's behavior and its habitat is one of the richest sources of clues for what is processed in the animal's brain. For example, psychophysical study of bats established that they used echolocation to navigate the environment, and this knowledge served as an impetus to study the bat's brain for neuron's sensitive to frequencies near those emitted by the bat and to search for neuron's selective to distortions attributable to Doppler shift (e.g., O'Neill & Suga, 1982). The consideration of the frog's habitat is evident in Lettvin's classic paper describing "bug detectors" in the optic tract of the frog (Lettvin, Maturana, McColloch, & Pitts, 1959).

Classic psychophysics measures sensory and discrimination thresholds. These measurements have been useful for exploring differences between sensory and discrimination thresholds in neurons versus the individual (e.g., Talbot, Darian-Smith, Kornhuber, & Mountcastle, 1968; reviewed in Parker & Newsome, 1998). Such information is useful to the investigator in establishing the relationships between neural and individual performance. Classic psychophysics has also been useful in characterizing the range over which neurons are sensitive. Thus, for example, psychophysics is useful for characterizing the spatial and temporal characteristics of visual neurons. Classic psychophysics has been relatively poor, however, in providing heuristics for discovering trigger features in neurons. The main purpose has been to provide a quantitative analysis of neurons that have already been characterized.

A different psychophysics has emerged since the 1960s. The "new" psychophysics has its roots in gestalt psychology (especially Kaffka & Lewin; reviewed in Murphy & Kovach, 1972) and was best articulated by James Gibson (1950, 1966, 1977). In contrast with classic psychophysics, which has its psychological roots in the constructivist psychology of Wilhelm Wundt, Gibson's stance was that the environment was a particularly rich source of information. The environment was sufficiently rich that the senses alone could drive perception; they did not need to be combined with memory or inference (the constructivist stance). Gibson believed that the task of psychology was to show that the world was filled with "higher-order" variables, and it was this sensitivity to such variables that drove perception directly. This point is well stated by the title of a paper by William Mace regarding Gibson's approach, "Ask Not What's Inside Your Head, Ask What Your Head Is Inside Of" (Mace, 1977). For neurophysiology, this perspective was important because it provided investigators with many different clues about what kinds of stimuli neurons might be sensitive to. Gibson's analyses and influence in showing the importance of optic flow during locomotion (1950, 1966; Gibson, Olum, & Rosenblatt, 1955) have proven useful in evaluating areas of visual cortex that appear specialized for supporting visually guided locomotion (e.g., Motter & Mountcastle, 1981; Rauschecker, Von Granau, & Poulin, 1987) and for facilitating the extraction of structure from motion in other cortical areas (e.g., Bradley, Chang, & Andersen, 1998). Gibson's perspective of searching for higher-order variables to explain perception is evident in Sussman's chapter (chapter 2 of this volume) showing how sophisticated analyses of speech utterances (the proximal stimulus) provide a useful metric for solving the noninvariance problem in speech perception.

Psychology/artificial intelligence. From different perspectives, each of these disciplines has focused attention on what a brain should be doing. Psychology has provided the conceptual foundations for what the mind does and shapes our expectations about what individual neurons might encode. Artificial intelligence (AI) has forced us to approach perception and action as computational problems. In so doing, AI has brought a rigor to neuroscience that would probably be otherwise absent. AI has done neuroscience another great favor by pointing out the real problem in understanding that the brain is not cataloguing that a neuron is sensitive to this or sensitive to that, but that understanding means that there is an algorithmic basis for *how* those properties emerge (discussed below; see Marr 1982).

It is no secret that psychology as a discipline emerged from psychology (e.g., even into the 1970s, the major neuroscience textbook was R. F. Thompson's *Foundations of Physiological Psychology*). Long before anyone struck an electrode into the brain, the idea of mechanical solutions to mind was already present. René Decartes was familiar with the concept of the reflex and promoted the idea that animals (but importantly, not humans) were mechanical devices driven by reflexes, referring to them as *automata*. Psychology has historically been wedded to a constructivist approach in understanding perceptual processes. Perceptions are constructed from sensations (the proximal stimulus) combined with memory (or experience). Such an approach was warranted because it was believed that the sensations were equivocal by themselves and needed to be combined with some other process, be it memory or inference, to produce the percept. One certain consequence of this view is that perception is believed to be constructed from the simple properties to the complex, and few would argue that this does not dominate current zeitgeist in neuroscience.

Collectively, psychology and AI have helped us appreciate one of the major accomplishments of the brain, the ability to abstract perceptions and actions. Importantly, these abstractions exist as representations, but the algorithmic basis for these representations remains elusive and the great question of neuroscience and AI. A few examples of this abstract knowledge illustrate both the remarkable achievement and the problem. In visual perception, we can recognize a cup or even the same cup, when we see it from a distance, close up, no matter what portion of the visual field, what angles, the many shades of lighting, and even (within reason) if we occlude portions of the cup. Under all these conditions we perceive the same cup, which is remarkable because the image formed on the back of the retina (the proximal stimulus) is, in every case, different. Thus, more than a million different patterns on the retina produced the same percept. In psychology, this phenomenon has been known as stimulus generalization, size constancy, or structural invariance (Gibson, 1966). A similar example can be found in the auditory system, where if 50 people say the name "Chuck," the spectrogram (a "fingerprint" of sound presented as two-dimensional images encoding time and frequency) revealing the proximal stimulus is, in every case, different. Yet in every instance, I will hear the name "Chuck." The motor system has an equivalent abstract knowledge, often referred to as "motor equivalence." For example, I can write my name with my left hand (easy, because I'm left-handed), I can write my name with my right hand, and I can write my name by putting the pen between my teeth and still create legible letters. In all cases, I produced a replica of the letters of my name. I was able to do so because I "understood" what needed to be done and, in each case, tailored a specific motor program to produce the letters. Yet in each case, the kinematics (i.e., exactly which muscles move and when) were different. This "understanding" means that somewhere in my brain I had an abstraction (which exists as a representation) of what needed to be produced, independent of the musculature I engage to perform the program.

How this abstraction is constructed is a difficult problem and occupies much more time in AI than it does in neuroscience. This issue is described below when discussing the second barrier to the neuron doctrine, deciphering how receptive fields acquire their properties. A much simpler question for neuroscience is where such abstractions are represented. For several reasons, including data from brain-damage patients, investigators were able to find neurons in the inferotemporal region of cortex that apparently respond selectively to faces (e.g., Perrett, Heitanen, Oram, & Benson, 1992). These neurons possess sophisticated properties because they respond not only to faces from a frontal view, but also when the head is rotated. Thus, they encode abstract, "higher-order" properties that are not tied to retinal coordinates and, apparently, embody a deep understanding of the properties of objects as they change orientations and perspectives. That such cells exist tells us something about the brain: abstract properties can be embedded in single neurons. We do not need to have a million cells to account for all views of a person's face. Individual cells apparently have a deep-level "understanding" of the properties that constitute a face. Yet we have very little idea how that occurs. How these neurons acquire their properties is the second barrier to implementing the neuron doctrine.

"Dumb Luck." Finally, it would be dishonest to pretend that scientists strictly use logic to solve their problems. Sometimes there is no substitute for dumb luck. That most neurons in visual cortex were sensitive to stimulus orientation was discovered by accident. David Hubel and Tortsen Wiesel were trying characterize the response properties of visual cortical neurons using spots of light. Apparently, one of them dropped a piece of paper across the projector they were using, causing a dark edge to move through the receptive field with a particular orientation. The cell's discharge was spectacular (we can be thankful that the paper had close to the preferred orientation), prompting them to start testing all their neurons with bars and edges of different orientations. As a result, these investigators discovered orientation columns (Hubel & Wiesel, 1962) and used these insights to propose their "hierarchical" theory of visual perception (Hubel & Wiesel, 1965). These observations figured prominently into their receiving the Nobel Prize in Physiology or Medicine in 1981.

Barrier 2: Neurons Are Embedded in Complicated Circuits That We Do Not Understand

The neuron doctrine is a two-step process. For the first step, some barriers to characterizing receptive fields have just been described. The second step, understanding how the receptive fields acquired their properties, is probably even worse, because the nervous system is not conveniently arranged for us. Nearly all neurons are embedded in complex circuits that we do not really understand. In this section, some of the problems encountered in trying to understand how the receptive field properties emerge are described.

Computational architecture. There are a few good things to say about the computational architecture of the brain. One is that it is largely a massively parallel machine in which operations, at least in the early stages, are kept separate. Second, it appears the operations are done in multiple steps that are anatomically separate. Thus, in vision, inputs from the retina are passed to the lateral geniculate nucleus of the thalamus and are then passed to visual cortex, which then appears to disperse information to many places. Third, the early stages appear to have what are referred to as *coarse* coding, meaning that the neurons respond to a wide variety of stimuli. Coarse coding is replaced at later stages by *sparse* coding, meaning that the neurons become very selective to the events that trigger them. This transition of coarse to sparse coding invites the idea that computation is run in a serially progressive way, and that may well be true. The problems emerge when serious modeling begins. In fact, only relatively few properties can be accounted for. As an example, Hubel and Wiesel (1962) first suggested that the simple cells of visual cortex obtained their orientation selectivity as a result of combining inputs from the concentrically organized receptive fields observed in the lateral geniculate nucleus of the thalamus. Their idea is probably true. Yet even today we still do not possess an algorithmic basis for these neurons (Ferster & Miller, 2000). Thus, although anatomical arrangements and receptive field properties can suggest that an algorithmic basis will be straightforward, even the simple is elusive.

In reality, nearly all serially arranged parallel networks include significant cross-talk and feedback connections. The functional significance of these connections is poorly understood, making predictive serial relationships problematic. Trigger features are rarely constructed from linear combinations of their inputs. Most neurons are deeply embedded in complex circuitry that behaves nonlinearly, and we currently do not possess the algebraic understanding of how the inputs are combined. To make matters worse, many of these connections are dynamically weighted, such that what might be a strong input at one instant is essentially nonexistent the next. Having said that, there are a number of published models that can account for some of the behavior some of the time, especially when the system is seriously constrained (e.g., Fuhrmann, Segey, Markram, & Tsodyks, 2002). The rigor of AI has forced us to the reality that these models must be highly quantitative and exact. The goal of AI is to actually build machines that see, hear, talk and act. There is not much "wiggle room" for vague concepts. The machine must work. One lesson here is that "explanation" has a very specific meaning. There is an algorithmic basis for linking the properties of cell A to cell B. Thus, when cell A fires an action potential, its efficacy on cell B must be quantifiable. For a neuron that receives 20 or more inputs (this *is* reality), the efficacy of any of the inputs on the target neuron should be understood in the context of the other inputs to realize the output. If it seems like a complicated problem, it is. The chapter by Canavier, Lovejoy, Perla, and Shepard (chapter 3 of this volume) acquaints the reader with the formidable complexity yet potentially rich information available in the temporal dynamics of the spike train of a single neuron.

Algorithmic solutions to understanding receptive field properties. The description of the receptive field is the first step of the neuron doctrine. It is a necessary and important step, because it tells *what* properties are being extracted. As described above, description of the neuron's receptive field is by no means a simple task. Perhaps most frustrating is that it nearly requires one to already understand the operations of the brain before starting. The second step is to explain how these properties emerge from the circuits in which they are embedded. Describing receptive field properties alone is useful, as they offer us clues as to what parameters might be of interest to the brain. Description by itself, however, is phenomenon, not mechanism. Consider the extreme case in which one somehow managed to simultaneously record from every neuron in the brain. Understanding the brain would still be in the distant future because the algorithms or rules that could account for how the activity of one neuron relates to another to produce the behavior would have to emerge from this monstrous data set.

Description becomes mechanistic when the description includes the rules for how the receptive field properties are constructed. This problem is difficult, because understanding the construction of receptive field properties is generally not derived from simple serial and linear addition. Instead, nearly all circuits are embedded in complex circuits. Most success has been found among neurons near sensory surfaces where the properties are simpler, at the level of the musculature where the relation of output to muscle length is so transparent, and in simpler nervous systems. Explanations of receptive field properties can be described as *qualitative* or *quantitative* models. Qualitative and quantitative models differ in the degree to which they account for explaining receptive field properties. Qualitative models are descriptive, with no formal attempt to write algorithms that tie input to output. Quantitative models include formal algorithms that link antecedent conditions to subsequent behavior of the neuron. The distinction is actually quite simple. Quantitative models provide the blueprints for building a brain or brain module, qualitative models do not. Quantitative models "explain" behavior. Qualitative models vary in their explanatory capacities, but none provides explicit algorithms. It should come as no surprise that most models are qualitative, because they are much easier than quantitative models. Qualitative models can be little more than sampling neurons in a structure, noting the correlations of the neural activity to exogenous events and proposing a plausible model.

Quantitative models are difficult to construct because the vast majority of neurons are deeply embedded in complicated circuits. Although it may be true that basic brain design is a massively parallel, hierarchical machine, there exists sufficient cross talk and feedback to render algorithms based on serially processing tenuous at best. As with most success in describing receptive field properties, it should come as little surprise that nearly all the success in modeling has come from studying the properties of neurons close to the sensory surface, or close to the musculature.

Because AI's goal is to build a machine, there is little room for vague concepts; the machine either works or it does not work. Less-than-exact algorithms and even descriptions, however, are of heuristic value. Neuroscientists use them all the time. Qualitative models can lead us in the direction of developing quantitative models. Konishi (chapter 1 of this volume) has pursued a logical progression of experiments in deciphering how the owl localizes sound, from physics, to psychophysics, to the construction of maps of space based on intra-aural intensity or timing differences. Konishi's models have not arrived at the level of accounting for individual spikes, but they do give a good accounting of how neurons at one level account for properties at the next level. Quantitative models can be broken into "soft" and "hard" models depending on whether the analysis is based on actual characterization of the inputs or on models of the inputs that would account for the outputs. Barlow and Levick's (1965) description of the directional selectivity (described above) is a good example of a "soft" quantitative model. Their model was sufficiently quantitative that real electronic parts could be substituted to model and account for directional selectivity. They were unable to show, however, that the input elements onto the directional cell actually behaved as their model would suggest. The model appears to mimic the observed properties and, as such, "explains" the directional selectivity, because one can build such a circuit. The model, however, is "soft" in the sense that the actual states of the inputs were never measured. Soft quantitative models can also exist for elements at the motor end. Robinson (e.g., 1981) has brought a "systems analysis" perspective to neuroscience. In studying the oculomotor system, he has been able to write quantitative equations that accurately relate the activity of neurons to the animal's oculomotor behavior. Remarkably, he has shown how most of the neurons conform to a relatively simple equation relating eye position to activity. Thus, given the firing rate of a neuron, he can make a good estimate of eye position, and conversely, given eye position, he can make a good estimate of the firing rate of the neuron. Robinson's approach has also been applied to larger pieces of behavior, including application of systems analysis to the vestibulo-ocular reflex (Robinson, 1989). The vestibulo-ocular reflex is a relatively simple behavior that allows us to continue looking at something even when we move our heads. Signals from the inner ear detect changes in head position and generate signals to the oculomotor system that move the eyes exactly equal and opposite of the detected changes in head position.

Understanding abstract representations. Finally, there is the sticky issue of understanding abstract representations. As introduced above, both psychology and AI are aware of the need for abstract representation. Abstract here means that representations of perceptions and actions exist in the brain in a topological domain that is not as constrained as the simpler and more common topographical representations. Topology is a broad field of mathematics that studies relations between domains. A common-sense definition of a representation is that it is a likeness. Representations formally describe a relationship between two (or more) domains. All representations contain entities ("things," "stuff"), attributes, and relations. Topography is a special case of topology and is considered a first-order transformation. The rule of topography is adjacency; adjacent points on the representation correspond to adjacent points on that which is represented. Thus, for example, in the visual system, many early areas are described as retinotopic; that is, adjacent points in primary visual cortex correspond to adjacent points on the retina. (Guido, Ziburkus, & Lo, in chapter 5 of this volume, discuss developmental issues in establishing retinotopic maps.) At some point as we move into deeper into the brain—that is, more synapses removed from sensory surfaces—the receptive fields of individual neurons are become larger, trigger features are usually more selective for specific events (sparse coding), and one is hard-pressed to demonstrate topography. For both AI and neuroscience, the algorithmic basis for moving from a topographical to a topological domain remains the greatest single challenge to the success of the neuron doctrine.

REFERENCES

Barlow, H. B. (1972). Single units and sensation: A neuron doctrine for perceptual psychology? *Perception, 1,* 371–394.

Barlow, H. B. (1995). The neuron doctrine in perception. In M. S. Gazzaniga (Ed.), *The cognitive sciences* (pp. 415–435). Cambridge, MA: MIT Press.

Barlow, H. B., & Levick, W. R. (1965). The mechanism of directionally selective units in the rabbit's retina. *Journal of Physiology (London), 178,* 477–504.

Bradley, D. C., Chang, G. C., & Andersen, R. A. (1998). Encoding of three-dimensional structure-from-motion by primate area MT neurons. *Nature, 392,* 714–717.

Ferster, D., & Miller, K. D. (2000). Neural mechanisms of orientation selectivity in the visual cortex. *Annual Review of Neuroscience, 23,* 441–471.

Furhmann, G., Segev, I., Markram, H., & Tsodyks, M. (2002). Coding of temporal information by activity-dependent synapses. *Journal of Neurophysiology, 87,* 140–148.

Gibson, J. J. (1950). *The perception of the visual world.* Boston: Houghton Mifflin.

Gibson, J. J. (1966). *The senses considered as perceptual systems.* Boston: Houghton Mifflin.

Gibson, J. J. (1977). The theory of affordances. In R. E. Shaw and J. Bransford (Eds.), *Perceiving, acting and knowing.* Hillsdale, NJ: Lawrence Erlbaum.

Gibson, J. J., Olum, P., & Rosenblatt, F. (1955). Parallax and perspective during aircraft landings. *American Journal of Psychology, 68,* 372–385.

Hubel, D. H., & Wiesel, T. N. (1962). Receptive fields, binocular interactions and functional architecture in the cat's striate cortex. *Journal of Physiology (London), 160,* 106–154.

Hubel, D. H., & Wiesel, T. N. (1965). Receptive field and functional architecture in two nonstriate visual areas (18 and 19) of the cat. *Journal of Neurophysiology, 28,* 229–289.

Lettvin, J. Y., Maturana, H. R., McCulloch, W. S., & Pitts, W. H. (1959). What the frog's eye tells the frog's brain. *Proceedings of the Institute of Radio Engineers, 47,* 1940–1951.

Mace, W. M. (1977). James J. Gibson's strategy for perceiving: Ask not what's inside your head, but what your head's inside of. In

R. E. Shaw and J. Bransford (Eds.), *Perceiving, acting and knowing.* Hillsdale, NJ: Lawrence Erlbaum.

Marr, D. (1982). *Vision.* New York: Freeman.

Motter, B. C., & Mountcastle, V. B. (1981). The functional properties of the light-sensitive neurons of the posterior parietal cortex studied in waking monkeys: Foveal sparing and opponent vector organization. *Journal of Neuroscience, 1,* 3–26.

Murphy, G. & Kovach, J. K. (1972). *Historical introduction to modern psychology* (3rd ed.). New York: Harcourt, Brace Jovanovich.

O'Neill, W. E., & Suga, N. (1982). Encoding of target range and its representation in the auditory cortex of the mustached bat. *Journal of Neuroscience, 2,* 17–31.

Parker, A. J., & Newsome, A. J. (1998). Sense and the single neuron: Probing the physiology of perception. *Annual Review of Neuroscience, 21,* 227–277.

Perrett, D. I., Heitanen, J. K., Oram, M. W., & Benson, P. J. (1992). Organization and function of cells responsive to faces in the temporal cortex. *Philosophical Transactions of the Royal Society London [Biology], 335,* 31–38.

Rauschecker, J. P., Von Granau, M. W., & Poulin, C. (1987). Centrifugal organization of directional preferences in the cat's lateral suprasylvian visual cortex and its relation to flow field processing. *Journal of Neuroscience, 7,* 943–958.

Robinson, D. A. (1981). The use of control systems analysis in the neurophysiology of eye movements. *Annual Review of Neuroscience, 4,* 463–503.

Robinson, D. A. (1989). Integrating with neurons. *Annual Review of Neuroscience, 12,* 33–45.

Talbot, W. H., Darian-Smith, I., Kornhuber, H. H., & Mountcastle, V. B. (1968). The sense of flutter-vibration: Comparison of the human capacity with response patterns of mechanoreceptive afferents from the monkey hand. *Journal of Neurophysiology, 31,* 301–334.

Tanji, J., & Shima, K. (1994). Role of supplementary motor area cells in planning several movements ahead. *Nature, 371,* 413–416.

5

Synaptic Plasticity in the Developing Visual Thalamus

William Guido, Jokubas Ziburkus, and Fu-Sun Lo
Department of Cell Biology and Anatomy and the Neuroscience Center of Excellence
Louisiana State University Health Sciences Center
New Orleans, LA

A major and enduring question in neuroscience is to understand the cellular mechanisms underlying the establishment and refinement of synaptic connectivity between developing sense organs and their central targets. Since the 1980s the mammalian retinogeniculate pathway has served as an important model for demonstrating how precise patterns of synaptic connections are formed and the manner in which patterned activity shapes them (Cramer & Sur, 1995; Erzurumlu & Guido, 1996; Goodman & Shatz, 1993; Shatz, 1990, 1996). This chapter reviews work in a rodent model of visual development to examine how retinal inputs from the two eyes undergo an activity-dependent period of synaptic remodeling to form adultlike patterns of connectivity in the lateral geniculate nucleus (LGN) of the dorsal thalamus. Color slides for this chapter can be found on the accompanying CD-ROM.

ANATOMICAL ORGANIZATION OF THE DEVELOPING RETINOGENICULATE PATHWAY

The mammalian visual system comprises highly ordered topographic maps. A distinguishing feature of these maps is the segregation of inputs from the two eyes at both the thalamic and cortical level (slide 1). Ganglion cells of each retina project in an ordered fashion to the LGN of the dorsal thalamus. Only those axons from the nasal region of retina, however, cross at the optic chiasm. Those from the temporal retina remain uncrossed and project to the ipsilateral LGN. Once in the LGN, retinal axons from each eye terminate into separate eye specific layers or domains. LGN projection neurons then send their axons to layer IV of visual cortex, where they too segregate. In some species, such as the cat and primate, thalamocortical axons terminate in alternating eye-specific bands or ocular dominance columns.

In the case of the rodent animal model under study, the Long Evans hooded rat, retinal projections from the two eyes form eye-specific domains in LGN rather than layers (Figure 5-1A–C, slide 2A–C) (Cowey & Perry, 1979; Lund, Lund, & Wise, 1978; Reese, 1988; Reese & Cowey, 1983; Reese & Jeffery, 1983). A closer look reveals (Figure 5-1B, slide 2B) that axons from the nasal retina as well as those representing the upper visual field of the temporal retina cross at the optic chiasm and project to the lateral and ventral regions in LGN (Figure 5-1A and B, slide 2A and B). These pro-

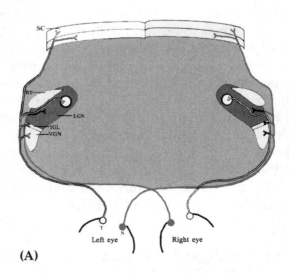

(A)

Figure 5-1. Pattern of retinal axon segregation in the LGN of the pigmented rat. (A) Diagram showing retinofugal projections. Axons from temporal regions of retina (*white*) project ipsilaterally and terminate as a small patch in the anterior-medial region of LGN. Axons from temporal regions of retina (*gray*) project contralaterally, crossing at the optic chiasm and terminating in a large ventral lateral region of LGN. (Adapted from Sefton & Dreher, 1995.)

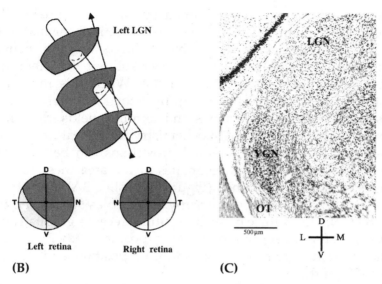

Figure 5-1. (continued). (B) Detailed view of retinal projections in LGN. Axons from the lower temporal "crescent" of retina (*white*) compose the uncrossed pathway. The remaining temporal region and the nasal aspect of retina (*gray*) compose the crossed pathway. In the coronal plane, the uncrossed projection approximates a cylinder that courses through the LGN. (Adapted from Reese & Jeffery, 1983.) (C) A coronal section of the dorsal lateral thalamus showing the LGN. Cells are visualized by a thionin nissl substance stain. The lateral geniculate nucleus (LGN), ventral geniculate nucleus (VGN), and the optic tract (OT) are readily discerned. The rodent LGN lacks an obvious lamination pattern, which in other species such as the ferret and cat partitions the LGN into eye-specific layers. Abbreviations: SC: superior colliculus; RT: reticular nucleus; LGN: lateral geniculate nucleus; IGL: intrageniculate leaflet; VGN: ventral geniculate nucleus; T: temporal; N: nasal; D:dorsal; V: ventral; L: lateral; M: medial.

jections occupy as much as 85% of the area in LGN. Retinal axons representing the lower visual field of temporal retina (i.e., the "temporal crescent") do not cross at the optic chiasm, but remain uncrossed and project ipsilaterally into the dorsal and medial anterior two-thirds of the nucleus (Figure 5-1A and B, slide 2A and B). These uncrossed projections form a cylinder through LGN and occupy about 15% of the total area in LGN.

Remarkably, this form of eye-specific patterning is not present during early development but emerges during early postnatal life (Jeffery, 1984). Initially, retinal arbors from the two eyes share common terminal space in LGN, and then, over a period of weeks, they segregate to form well-defined eye-specific domains. This present study examined the time course of retinogeniculate axon segregation in the developing rat by labeling axons and their terminal fields with the anterograde tracer subunit B cholera toxin (CTB) (Angelucci, Clasca, & Sur, 1996). When this material is injected into one eye, it is taken up by retinal ganglion cells and transported through their axons and terminal fields. By using a peroxidase based immunocytochemistry to reveal the axonal transport of CTB in LGN, retinal projections can be visualized (Figure 5-2A, slide 3A) and estimates of the area these terminal fields occupy can be obtained (Figure 5-2B, slide 3A). At birth, the uncrossed retinal projections occupy as much as 90% of the total area in LGN. This diffuse projection pattern recedes gradually during the first few weeks of life so that by postnatal day 21, the ipsilateral projection retracts to its adultlike position and occupies about 15% of the LGN.

FUNCTIONAL ORGANIZATION OF THE DEVELOPING RETINOGENICULATE PATHWAY

The gradual refinement of the uncrossed retinal pathway suggests that a significant amount of synaptic remodeling occurs in the LGN during the first three weeks of postnatal life. To explore the functional implications associated with such changes, the physiology and pharmacology underlying the synaptic responses of developing LGN cells were examined. Used was a unique in vitro isolated brain stem recording preparation. This preparation is especially suited for the study of synaptic transmission because unlike a conventional slice preparation, in the isolated brain stem preparation, retinal axons innervating the LGN as well as the intrinsic geniculate circuitry remain intact. Figure 5-3 and slide 4 depict the preparation and the basic experimental approach. The rodent brain is surgically excised, cut in half along the midline axis, and placed into a well of a temperature-controlled in vitro recording chamber. The brain stem, midbrain, and thalamus are exposed by surgically removing the forebrain (i.e., neocortex, hippocampus, and striatum). The preparation is then submerged and perfused continuously with a warmed and oxygenated artificial cerebrospinal fluid. Stimulating electrodes are placed on the surface of the optic nerves, and an intracellular recording electrode is inserted into LGN. By electrically stimulating the optic nerves,

(A)

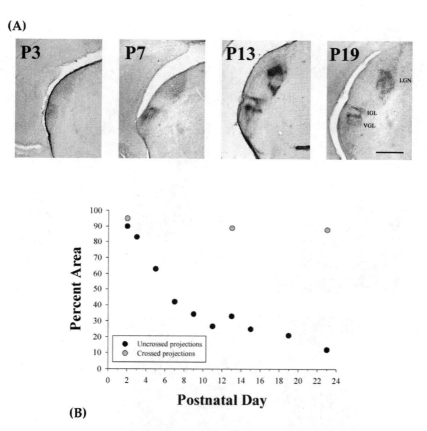

(B)

Figure 5-2. Pattern of retinogeniculate projections in the developing rat revealed by the anterograde transport of the subunit B of cholera toxin (CTB). (A) Coronal sections of the lateral thalamus (left to right) at postnatal (P) days 3, 7, 13, and 19 showing the developmental changes in the size and breadth of the uncrossed retinogeniculate projection in LGN after a left-eye injection of CTB. Note also the labeling in the intrageniculate leaflet (IGL) and the ventral geniculate nucleus (VLG). Visualization of anterogradely transported CTB is accomplished by peroxidase-based immunocytochemistry. The scale bar is 500 μm. (B) Plot showing the total area in LGN occupied by the uncrossed (*black symbols*) and crossed retinal (*gray symbols*) projections at various postnatal ages. Measurements are based on a rostral to caudal series of 40-μm-thick sections through LGN.

synaptic activity in LGN cells in the form of excitatory (EPSP) and inhibitory (IPSP) postsynaptic potentials can be evoked. It is also possible to apply a variety of receptor antagonists to the bath and determine the underlying pharmacology of these responses. Finally, by using dye-filled electrodes during our intracellular recordings, cells can be visualized and structure-function correlations can be established.

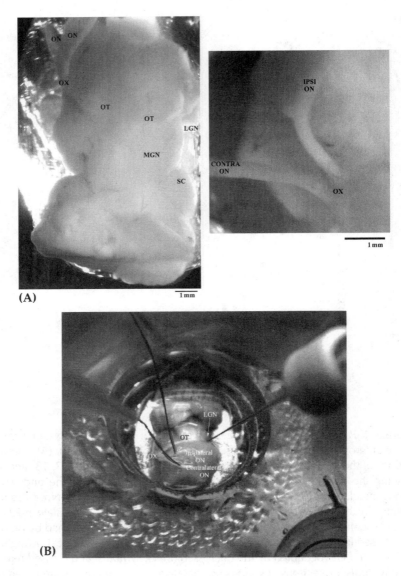

Figure 5-3. The isolated brain stem preparation and experimental approach. (A) *Left:* Dorsal view of the preparation, showing the optic nerves (ON), optic chiasm (OX), optic tract (OT), medial geniculate nucleus (MGN), lateral geniculate nucleus (LGN) of the dorsal thalamus, and the midbrain structure, the superior colliculus (SC). *Right:* High-power view showing the optic nerves (ON) and optic chiasm (OX). (B) Photograph of the preparation in the temperature-controlled recording chamber. It is kept submerged and perfused continuously with artificial cerebrospinal fluid. Stimulating electrodes are positioned in each optic nerve and a recording electrode into the LGN. Electrical stimulation of the optic nerves activates retinal axons and evokes synaptic activity in LGN.

The rodent LGN contains two morphologically distinct cell types (slides 5 and 8), thalamic projection neurons or relay cells that have complex radially oriented dendritic trees and axons that project to layer IV of visual cortex, and intrinsic interneurons, with processes that span large regions of the LGN but reside exclusively within the nucleus (Parnavelas, Mounty, Bradford, & Lieberman, 1977; Sefton & Dreher, 1995; Webster & Rowe, 1984). In a mature relay cell, retinal stimulation commonly evokes an excitatory post-synaptic potential (EPSP) that is followed by inhibitory postsynaptic activity (IPSP) (Figure 5-4B and C and slide 6). These EPSP/IPSP pairs reveal that retinal axons make excitatory connections with relay cells (Scharfman, Lu, Guido, Adams, & Sherman, 1990). Retinal axons also possess collaterals that form excitatory connections with neighboring interneurons that in turn form a feed-forward inhibitory connection with relay cells (slide 6) (Crunelli, Haby, Jassik-Gerschenfeld, Leresche, & Pirchio, 1988; Lindström, 1982). From a functional standpoint, these EPSP/IPSP pairs underlie the basis of retinogeniculate signal transmission (Sherman & Guillery, 1996). When EPSPs depolarize the membrane potential to a level that exceeds spike threshold (about –45 mV), action potentials ensue. When EPSPs fail to depolarize the membrane potential above the level of spike threshold, however, signaling ceases. IPSP activity helps set the overall gain of signaling by hyperpolarizing the membrane potential and decreasing the probability of action potential firing.

These features of retinogeniculate signal transmission are not present during early postnatal development. Instead, the bulk of synaptic responses (70%) at early ages are purely excitatory (Figure 5-4A, slide 6A). Pharmacology experiments indicate excitatory responses are mediated by glutamate receptor activation and involve the coincident activation of two receptor subtypes, conventionally classified as N-methyl-D-aspartate (NMDA) and non-NMDA or AMPA (Chen & Regehr, 2000; Scharfman et al., 1990). Although both receptors use glutamate as a neurotransmitter, they differ in their voltage dependency, ion selectivity, and affinity for certain agonists and antagonists. The non-NMDA component of the EPSP is a conventional Na^{2+}/K^+ conductance that has a fast-rising depolarization with an amplitude that decreases with membrane depolarization. The NMDA component of the EPSP is a slowly rising, long-lasting depolarization that actually increases in amplitude with membrane depolarization, due to a voltage-dependent Mg^{2+} ion blockade that exists near resting

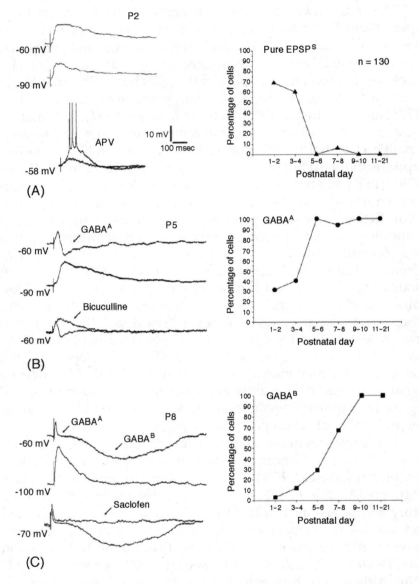

Figure 5-4. Synaptic transmission in the developing LGN. Synaptic responses of LGN cells are evoked by electrical stimulation of the optic tract. The accompanying graphs plot the incidence of pure EPSPs (A), GABA$_A$ (B), and GABA$_B$ IPSPs (C) as a function of age. (A) Examples of pure EPSPs recorded at postnatal day 2. *Top*: EPSPs recorded at –60 mV and –90 mV. The EPSP at –60 mV has a long decay time, underscoring the presence of a large NMDA component. *Bottom*: EPSPs before and after the bath application of the NMDA antagonist (15 µM) APV. The late component is abolished, thereby reducing the amplitude and duration of the EPSP and preventing it from reaching spike threshold. The incidence of EPSP activity is 65–70% at early ages. (B) Examples of EPSPs *(continues)*

coupled with IPSP activity at P5. *Top*: At –60 mV, the EPSP is followed by a short-duration IPSP. At –90 mV, the IPSP reverses, suggesting it is mediated by a Cl⁻ conductance. *Bottom*: Postsynaptic activity before and after the bath application of the GABA$_A$ antagonist bicuculline (10 μM). The early IPSP is abolished, indicating that it is mediated by the activation of GABA$_A$ receptors. (C) Example of EPSP/IPSP activity at P8. *Top*: At –60 mV, a delayed and longer-lasting IPSP emerges. At –100mV, this late IPSP reverses, suggesting that it is mediated by K⁺ conductance. Postsynaptic activity is shown before and after the application of the GABA$_B$ antagonist saclofen (100 μM). At –70 mV, the late IPSP is blocked by saclofen, indicating that it is mediated by the activation of GABA$_B$ receptors. Inhibitory activity emerges as early as P3, but the full complement of GABA$_A$ and GABA$_B$ IPSP activity does not appear until P10.

membrane levels. To discern NMDA responses from non-NMDA ones, one must record at depolarized membrane levels to relieve the Mg^{2+} ion blockade or apply specific NMDA antagonists such as APV. Experiments of this sort reveal that a large component of the EPSP in developing LGN cells is composed of NMDA activity (Chen & Regehr, 2000; Ramoa & McCormick, 1994). The unique voltage dependency of NMDA receptors figures prominently in development because it allows for an influx of Ca^{2+} ions (along with a Na^{+2} influx and K⁺ efflux) during periods of heightened neural activity. It is the activity-dependent sequestration of Ca^{2+} that triggers a cascade of intracellular signaling events responsible for the eventual consolidation of adult patterns of connectivity (Constantine-Paton, Cline, & Debski, 1990; Cramer & Sur, 1995; Ghosh & Greenberg, 1995; Winder & Sweatt, 2001).

After the first few postnatal days of pure excitatory activity, inhibitory responses begin to emerge. The full complement of IPSP activity, however, is not evident until P10 (Figure 5-4B, slide 6B). Inhibitory responses are mediated by two types of GABA receptors. The first to appear is an early, fast-hyperpolarizing response and involves a Cl⁻ conductance through the GABA$_A$ receptor subtype (Crunelli, et al., 1988). This form of inhibitory activity reverses at membrane levels more negative than –80 mV (a point at which there is neither inward nor outward current flow and that corresponds to the Nernst potential for Cl⁻) and is blocked by the GABA$_A$ receptor antagonist bicuculline. These early fast GABA$_A$-mediated IPSPs also affect EPSP activity, often curtailing the late NMDA component of the excitatory response (Figure 5-4, slides 5 and 6). Another IPSP emerges near the end of the first week and involves a G-protein-activated K⁺ conductance through a GABA$_B$ receptor subtype (Crunelli et al., 1988). This response follows the $GABA_A$-mediated IPSP. It is slower and long-lasting, reverses at membrane levels more negative than –90 mV (the Nernst potential for K^+), and is blocked by the $GABA_B$ antagonist saclofen. These experiments indicate that excitatory and inhibitory synapses in LGN develop at different rates, with inhibitory ones maturing more slowly than excitatory ones (slide 7). The functional significance of this indication is not clear, but the delayed onset of inhibitory activity may promote an increased level of excitatory postsynaptic events (e.g., NMDA and Ca^{2+} channel activity) that have been implicated in synaptic remodeling (Lo, Ziburkus, & Guido, 2002; Ramoa & McCormick, 1994).

In addition to these age-related changes in postsynaptic receptor function, changes in the circuitry underlying synaptic transmission in LGN were noted. For example, the transient retinal inputs, particularly those that comprise the uncrossed retinal projection, actually make functional connections with LGN cells. As one would expect from the eye-specific patterning in the adult LGN, mature relay cells are monocular, receiving input from one or the other eye. Given the diffuse nature of early retinal projections, however, it is conceivable that immature LGN cells are binocular, receiving input from both eyes. Indeed, there is a high incidence of binocular responses (70%) during early development (Figure 5-5, slide 8). When recording in regions of the LGN that in the adult receive input exclusively from the contralateral eye (crossed retinal projections), separate and distinct EPSPs are readily evoked by stimulation of either optic nerve (Figure 5-5A, slide 8A). Often, especially between P7 and P14, binocularly mediated EPSP/IPSP pairs are observed (Figure 5-5C, slide 8C, top trace). Between P14 and 21, however, when uncrossed retinal projections are receding, the incidence of excitatory binocular responses is substantially reduced, and the majority of cells (71%) are monocular (Figure 5-5C, slide 8C, middle trace). Interestingly, what remains in many of these cells is a binocularly mediated inhibitory response (Figure 5-5C, slide 8C, bottom trace). Binocular inhibitory responses seem to arise from interneurons that receive input from one eye and then inhibit relay cell activity from the other eye (Alhsén, Lindström, & Lo, 1985). Coupling these current observations in the rat with those documented in the cat (Alhsén et al., 1985; Guido, Tumosa, & Spear, 1989) and monkey (Schroeder, Tenke, Arezzo, & Vaughan, 1990) suggests that such interactions are a fundamental feature of geniculate circuitry.

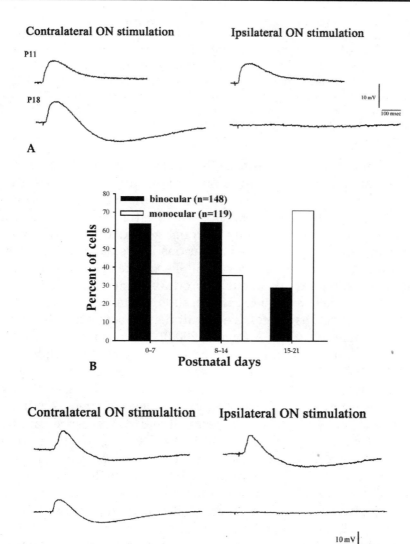

Figure 5-5. Age-related changes in binocular and monocular responses in the developing LGN. (A) Synaptic responses evoked by contralateral (*left*) and ipsilateral (*right*) optic nerve (ON) stimulation. At early ages, activation of either ON evokes EPSP activity. This cell receives binocular input. At later ages, contralateral ON stimulation evokes an EPSP/IPSP pair, but ipsilateral ON stimulation fails to yield a response. This cell receives monocular input. (B) Summary plot showing the incidence of binocular and monocular excitatory responses at P0–P7, P8–P14, and P15–P21. (C) Examples of binocular excitatory *(continues)*

and inhibitory interactions in the developing LGN. *Top:* Example of a binocularly innervated LGN cell. Stimulation of contralateral and ipsilateral ON evokes an EPSP that is followed by IPSP activity. *Middle:* Example of a mature, monocularly innervated cell in which contralateral ON stimulation evokes a response. *Bottom:* Example of a mature cell in which contralateral ON stimulation evokes an EPSP/IPSP pair and ipsilateral ON stimulation only an IPSP. All responses are recorded at –65 mV.

Another transient feature in the development of retinogeniculate transmission is the prevalence of synaptic responses that reflect the convergence of multiple retinal ganglion cell inputs onto a single LGN cell (Figure 5-6, slide 9). To estimate the number of retinal inputs converging onto a signal geniculate cell, the optic nerves are electrically shocked at various levels of stimulus intensity and the amplitudes of evoked EPSPs are measured. A progressive increase in stimulus intensity produces a stepwise increase in EPSP amplitude (Figure 5-6A and B, slide 9A and B). This relation is taken to reflect the successive recruitment of active inputs innervating a single cell (Chen & Regehr, 2000). Between P0 and P7, cells receive at least 3 to 6 inputs from each eye (Figure 5-6C, slide 9C). Thus, a single LGN cell can receive as many as 12 retinal inputs. Indeed, these estimates may be conservative. In mice, developing LGN cells receive as many as 20 inputs (Chen & Regehr, 2000). By P15 to P21, however, the degree of retinal convergence rapidly declines (Figure 5-6C, slide 9C), so that LGN cells, like their adult counterparts, receive input from just 1 to 3 retinal ganglion cells (Chen & Regehr, 2000; Mastronarde, 1987; Ursey, Reppas, & Reid, 1999). The most significant loss of inputs is among those that originate from the ipsilateral eye (uncrossed retinal projections). In fact, by P15 to P21, there is almost a total elimination of inputs from this eye (Figure 5-6C, slide 9C). Of course, this result is entirely consistent with the age-related loss of binocular response properties noted earlier. The decrease in inputs may also help explain the dynamic changes in receptive field structure in developing LGN cells. Immature LGN cells have very large, irregularly shaped receptive fields and poorly organized on- and off-subregions (Tavazoie & Reid, 2000). In contrast, mature LGN cells have much smaller receptive fields with a highly concentric antagonistic center-surround organization (Sherman & Guillery, 1996). Finally, it is important to note that the loss of binocular input coupled with the reduction in retinal convergence occurs during the most active phase of retinogeniculate axon segregation (slide 10).

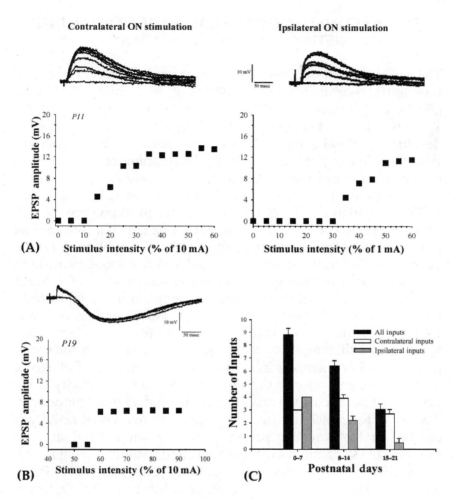

Figure 5-6. Retinal convergence in the developing LGN. (A and B) Examples of synaptic responses and corresponding amplitude by stimulus intensity plots for a binocular (A) and monocular cell (B). Synaptic responses are evoked by stimulating retinal fibers at progressively higher levels of stimulus intensity. An increase in stimulus intensity produces a stepwise increase in EPSP amplitude. Steps reflect the successive recruitment of additional retinal inputs. The binocular cell (A) receives a total of seven inputs and the monocular one (B) just a single input from the contralateral retina. (C) Summary graph plotting means and standard errors for total number of inputs (*black*), contralateral inputs (*white*), and ipsilateral ones (*gray*) for LGN cells at P0–P7, P8–P14, and P15–P21.

EARLY RETINAL ACTIVITY SHAPES THE DEVELOPING RETINOGENICULATE PATHWAY

The establishment of orderly connections in LGN has been attributed to the coordinated firing patterns of developing retinal ganglion cells (Cramer & Sur, 1995; Shatz, 1990, 1996; Wong, 1999). This view is based on studies describing the firing properties of developing retinal ganglion cells and the consequences associated with the silencing of retinal activity. Developing retinal ganglion cells have very complex dendritic fields and are equipped with a full complement of membrane properties needed to generate action potentials (Liets & Chalupa, 2001; Skailora, Scoobey, & Chalupa, 1993; Wang, Ratto, Bisti, & Chalupa, 1997). Even before photoreceptors are operational, aggregates of neighboring retinal ganglion cells are synaptically coupled and fire spontaneously in rhythmic bursts of activity (2–6 sec in duration at rates of 7–50 Hz every 30–100 sec) that traverse across the retina in wavelike fashion (Maffei & Galli-Resta, 1990; Miester, Wong, Baylor, & Shatz, 1991; Wong, Miester, & Shatz, 1993; Wong & Oakley, 1996). The spontaneous discharges of retinal ganglion cells are sufficient to generate action potentials in LGN cells (Mooney, Penn, Gallego, & Shatz, 1996), and prior to eye opening, this form of activity is the primary (if not exclusive) driving force behind all thalamic activity (Weliky & Katz, 1999). When early spontaneous retinal activity is blocked or the wavelike patterns severely altered, retinal axon arbors in LGN maintain a diffuse projection pattern, having abnormally widespread terminal arborizations (Chapman, 2000; Penn, Riquelme, Fuller, & Shatz, 1998; Shatz & Stryker, 1988; Sretavan, Shatz, & Stryker, 1988). As a result, retinal axons fail to segregate into eye-specific domains. LGN cells are also affected by activity blockade, showing an increase in dendritic spine density (Dalva, Ghosh, & Shatz, 1994), anomalous receptive field properties (Dubin, Stark, & Archer, 1986), abnormal patterns of arborization in visual cortex (Hermann & Shatz, 1995), and a disruption in the development of NMDA receptor subunit composition (Ramoa & Prusky, 1997).

Perhaps the most celebrated model for explaining how the activity of immature neurons can form orderly connections is the Hebb (1949) synapse. In this model (Figure 5-7, slide 11), high levels of coincident activity between pre- and postsynaptic elements lead to a strengthening and consolidation of synapses. A corollary of this basic rule is that low levels of activity result in synapse

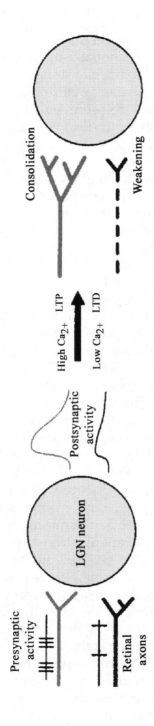

Figure 5-7. Modified Hebbian model of synaptic plasticity. Schematic showing how retinal activity leads to long-term changes in synaptic strength and the eventual stabilization of retinogeniculate connections. Shown are two retinal axons competing for terminal space on a single target neuron in LGN. Retinal spike activity is illustrated above each input as simple spike trains. Heightened retinal activity evokes large EPSP activity in the LGN neuron. The coincident pairing of heightened pre- and postsynaptic activity leads to a long-term potentiation (LTP) in subsequent synaptic activity. Accompanying these events is a large Ca^{2+} influx through the NMDA iontophore and/or voltage-gated Ca^{2+} channels. Increased levels of intracellular Ca^{2+} trigger a series of signaling events that leads to the strengthening and eventual consolidation of a synapse. On the other hand, low levels of retinal activity evoke smaller EPSP activity, weaker and somewhat asynchronous pairing of pre- and postsynaptic activity, a long-term depression (LTD) of subsequent synaptic activity, and less Ca^{2+} influx. Low levels of intracellular Ca^{2+} activate a separate set of signaling events that results in a weakening and eventual elimination of a synapse.

weakening and elimination (Bear, Cooper, & Ebner, 1987; Constantine-Paton et al., 1990; Cramer and Sur, 1995; Stent, 1973). A proposed substrate for activity-dependent remodeling is based on forms of synaptic plasticity first demonstrated in the hippocampus, in which the degree of frequency pairing between pre- and postsynaptic elements leads to a long-term potentiation (LTP) or depression (LTD) in synaptic strength (Bear & Malenka, 1994; Dudek & Bear, 1993; Kirkwood, Dudek, Aizenman, & Bear, 1993). In this model, NMDA receptor activation is needed for the induction of changes in synaptic efficacy (Collingridge, 1992). The voltage dependency of NMDA receptors enables them to act as "coincident detectors." That is, Ca^{2+} entry through NMDA receptors only occurs when there is sufficient depolarization. A large increase in the intracellular concentration of Ca^{2+} (high levels of NMDA receptor activation) triggers a distinct signaling cascade that leads to the strengthening of co-active elements. Modest or low levels of intracellular Ca^{2+} (low levels of NMDA receptor activation) trigger a different signaling cascade that leads to the weakening and eventual loss of less active, asynchronous ones. In the developing neocortex, there is evidence indicating that LTP and LTD exist and that an influx of Ca^{2+} through NMDA receptors contributes to the formation of orderly connections (Kirkwood & Bear, 1994a, 1994b). Such long-term modifications in synaptic strength may therefore embody the synaptic rearrangements occurring during the time of retinogeniculate axon segregation, when afferents from the two eyes are competing for common postsynaptic sites. To test for this possibility, the isolated brain stem preparation was used, and the synaptic responses of LGN cells before and after high-frequency stimulation (HFS) of a single optic nerve were examined (Figure 5-8, slide 12). The tetanus protocol, which consists of six 1-sec trains of 50-Hz stimulation delivered every 30 sec for 3 minutes, is designed to mimic (at least in the temporal domain) the intrinsic firing patterns of developing retinal ganglion cells (Wong et al., 1993; Wong & Oakley, 1996). This form of stimulation produces robust changes in synaptic strength (Figure 5-7, slide 12). In cells that receive input from the contralateral eye (crossed retinal projections), HFS of the contralateral optic nerve produces a long-term increase (150%) in the amplitude of EPSPs evoked by a single shock. This change is referred to as homosynaptic potentiation because the increase in synaptic strength occurs along the tetanized (or conditioned) pathway (Malenka & Siegelbaum, 2001). In cells that receive input from the two eyes,

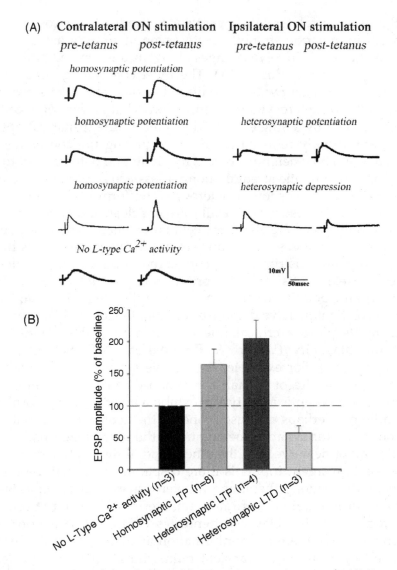

Figure 5-8. Activity dependent modifications in synaptic strength. (A) Examples of synaptic responses in four different LGN cells recorded before (pretetanus, *left*) and after (posttetanus, *right*) high-frequency stimulation of the contralateral optic nerve (ON). Synaptic responses along the tetanized pathway exhibit a homosynaptic potentiation. In some binocular cells, the synaptic responses recorded along the untetanized pathway exhibit a heterosynaptic potentiation and for others a heterosynaptic depression. The lack of L-type Ca^{2+} activity during tetanus resulted in no change in synaptic strength. Representative responses are obtained 5 minutes before and 10 minutes after tetanus. (B) Bar graph showing the posttetanus (at 10 minutes) changes in EPSP amplitude for the different groups. Values depict means and standard errors. Changes in synaptic strength are assessed using the Wilcoxon matched pairs signed rank test.

HFS of the contralateral optic nerve also produces heterosynaptic changes in synaptic strength. Heterosynaptic effects are considered as those that involve changes along an untetanized pathway (Malenka & Siegelbaum, 2001). The most compelling effect and one that is consistent with a modified Hebbian model of synaptic plasticity is of heterosynaptic depression. That is, for some cells, EPSPs evoked by a single shock delivered to the ipsilateral optic nerve are actually reduced (50%) by tetanizing the contralateral optic nerve. Thus, heightened activity along one pathway led to a reduction in synaptic strength along a less active pathway. Some cells, however, also show a heterosynaptic form of potentiation. The reasons for these varied results are not clear, and on this point one can only speculate about the cellular mechanisms underlying the observed changes in synaptic strength. One possibility is that the location and distribution of convergent inputs along the dendrites of relay cells play important roles in determining the strength and polarity of changes in synaptic strength (slide 14). Some investigators have demonstrated that the location of convergent inputs plays a critical role in determining the polarity of synaptic plasticity (Engert & Bonhoeffer, 1997; Schuman & Madison, 1994). For example, an inactive synapse that is within ~70 μm of the site of a tetanized synapse can benefit from the spread of presynaptic activity and exhibit a heterosynaptic form of potentiation. Perhaps this case is one for the heterosynaptic potentiation noted for synapses belonging to the untetanized pathway (ipsilateral optic nerve). On the other hand, if the relative distance between convergent inputs is more disparate, there will be little cooperativity among them, and a heterosynaptic depression will prevail. Although it is clear that retinal terminals cluster at proximal regions of the relay cell dendrites (Wilson, Friedlander, & Sherman, 1984), there is no information available about the location and distribution of transient retinal inputs (i.e., those originating from the ipsilateral eye). Thus, the location and distribution of contralateral and ipsilateral retinal inputs may be critical factors in predicting the amplitude and polarity of heterosynaptic changes in synaptic strength.

Another aspect of these results worth noting is the underlying pharmacology. Many examples of synaptic plasticity in the hippocampus and the neocortex seem to rely on NMDA receptor activation (Bear & Malenka, 1994; Constantine-Paton et al., 1990; Cramer & Sur, 1995). The plasticity observed in LGN, however, seems to rely on the activation of a high-threshold L-type Ca^{2+}

channel. For example, both homosynaptic and heterosynaptic forms of plasticity noted in LGN depend on the activation of a large, long-lasting plateaulike depolarization that is evoked during tetanus (Figure 5-9, slide 13). These depolarizations are mediated by high-threshold L-type Ca^{2+} channel activity triggered by a massive spatial and temporal summation of EPSPs (Lo, Ziburkus, & Guido, 2002). When this form of activity is prevented because the activation of L-type channels is prevented, either because it is

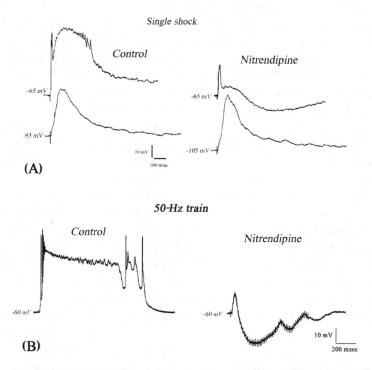

Figure 5-9. Plateau potentials in LGN. (A) Pharmacology of the plateau potential. At −65 mV, a single shock of the optic tract at high stimulus intensity evokes a large plateau depolarization (*control*). At a more hyperpolarized level (−93 mV), an identical form of stimulation fails to evoke a plateau potential, but results in a large postsynaptic response. In the presence of the L-type Ca^{2+} channel antagonist nitrendipine, the plateau potential is abolished, and what remains are an underlying EPSP and IPSP (nitrendipine). At −105 mV, a large postsynaptic potential is present, indicating that nitrendipine does not impede synaptic transmission. (B) A large long-lasting plateau potential is evoked by high-frequency stimulation (50 Hz). Nitrendipine, however, blocks the tetanus-evoked plateau potential. The tetanus-induced plateau potential is necessary for the induction of long-term changes in synaptic strength.

blocked pharmacologically or because the membrane potential is not sufficiently depolarized during teatnus, the HFS of the optic nerve fails to induce any changes in synaptic strength (Figure 5-8, slide 12). Thus, the activation of NMDA receptors need not be the sole source of Ca^{2+} during synaptic transmission, but a much larger and longer influx can occur via the activation of L-type Ca^{2+} channels (Budde, Munsch, & Pape, 1998). The Ca^{2+} influx associated with the synaptically evoked plateau potential could play an important role in the experience-dependent modification of the visual system, contributing to signaling events that underlie the stabilization of retinogeniculate connections. A role for L-type Ca^{2+} channels in synaptic plasticity has precedence. Activity in these channels can induce synaptic depression and potentiation in a number of structures including the hippocampus (Magee & Johnson, 1997), superior colliculus (Lo & Mize, 2000) and principal nucleus of the brain stem (Guido, Lo, & Erzurumlu, 2001). Another important consideration is the location of retinal synapses in relation to L-type Ca^{2+} channels (slide 14). Previous studies indicate that the L-type Ca^{2+} channels are unevenly distributed along the dendritic shafts of relay cells (Budde et al., 1998; Munsch, Budde, & Pape, 1997). Certainly, if a given set of retinal inputs clusters around a high concentration of L-type Ca^{2+} channels, it could lead to varied forms of synaptic plasticity. Finally, one must consider the temporal aspects of Ca^{2+} signaling. For example, the Ca^{2+} influx associated with the high-frequency activation of retinal afferents seems to persist for several seconds (Lo et al., 2002) and as a result may be paired with a synaptic responses evoked by the either the tetanized or untetanized pathway (Malenka & Siegelbaum, 2001). Clearly, more work needs to be done to explore these possibilities. Nonetheless, these experiments reveal that retinal activity can lead to long-term changes in synaptic strength and that some of these modifications are consistent with a Hebbian model of synaptic plasticity.

CONCLUSIONS

The retinogeniculate synapse undergoes a significant period of remodeling during early postnatal life. At birth, retinal axons from the two eyes share common terminal space in LGN. During the first three weeks of life, however, there is an age-related recession in the amount of terminal space occupied by the two eyes. By three weeks of age, the crossed and uncrossed retinal pathways segregate to form separate and distinct eye-specific domains, with the axons of uncrossed pathway occupying about 15% of the LGN. These structural changes also have functional correlates. At birth, excitatory synaptic responses prevail and most cells are binocularly innervated. There is also a high degree of retinal convergence such that a LGN single cell receives excitatory input from as many as 7 to 12 different retinal ganglion cells. During the time of retinogeniculate axon segregation (P5–P21), inhibitory responses emerge and LGN cells become monocularly innervated, losing the excitatory connections they initially made with uncrossed retinal projections. During this period of intense synaptic remodeling, changes in synaptic strength can be induced by the high-frequency stimulation of retinal fibers in a manner that approximates their spontaneous activity. These changes in synaptic strength, which are thought to herald the refinement of sensory connections, last several minutes and rely on the activation of the L-type species of voltage-gated Ca^{2+} channels. The polarity and magnitude of these changes vary. In most cases, however, they conform to a Hebbian model of activity-dependent synaptic plasticity.

ACKNOWLEDGMENTS

We thank Erick Green for his expert technical assistance in many phases of these projects and Dr. Reha Erzurumlu for his help in preparing and photographing the Dil labeled material. This study was supported by grants from the Whitehall Foundation and National Eye Institute (EY12716).

REFERENCES

Ahlsén, G., Lindström, S., & Lo, F. S. (1985). Interaction between inhibitory pathways to principal cells in the lateral geniculate nucleus of the cat. *Experimental Brain Research, 58,* 134–143.

Angelucci, A., Clasca, F., & Sur, M. (1996). Anterograde axonal tracing with the subunit B of cholera toxin: A highly sensitive immunohistochemical protocol for revealing fine axonal morphology in adult and neonatal brains. *Journal of Neuroscience Methods, 65,* 101–112.

Bear, M. F., Cooper, L. N., & Ebner, F. F. (1987). A physiological basis for a theory of synapse modification. *Science, 237,* 42–48.

Bear, M. F., & Malenka, R. C. (1994). Synaptic plasticity, LTP, and LTD. *Current Opinions in Neurobiology, 4,* 389–399.

Budde, T., Munsch, T., & Pape, H. C. (1998). Distribution of L-type calcium channels in rat thalamic neurons. *European Journal of Neuroscience, 10,* 586–597.

Chapman, B. (2000). Necessity for afferent activity to maintain eye-specific segregation in ferret lateral geniculate nucleus. *Science, 287,* 2479–2482.

Chen, C., & Regehr, W. G. (2000). Developmental remodeling of the retinogeniculate synapse. *Neuron, 28,* 955–966.

Collingridge, G. (1992). The mechanism of induction of receptor-dependent long-term potentiation in the hippocampus. *Experimental Physiology, 77,* 771–797.

Constantine-Paton, M., Cline, H. T., & Debski, E. (1990). Patterned activity, synaptic convergence, and the NMDA receptor in developing visual pathways. *Annual Review of Neuroscience, 13,* 129–154.

Cowey, A., & Perry, V. H. (1979). The projection of the temporal retina in rats, studied by retrograde transport of horseradish peroxidase. *Experimental Brain Research, 2,* 457–464.

Cramer, K. S., & Sur, M. (1995). Activity dependent remodeling of connections in the mammalian visual system. *Current Opinions in Neurobiology, 5,* 106–111.

Crunelli, V., Haby, M., Jassik-Gerschenfeld, D., Leresche, N., & Pirchio, M. (1988). Cl$^-$ and K$^+$ dependent inhibitory postsynaptic potentials evoked by interneurones of the rat lateral geniculate nucleus. *Journal of Physiology, 399,* 153–176.

Dalva, M. B., Ghosh, A., & Shatz, C. J. (1994). Independent control of dendritic and axonal form in the developing lateral geniculate nucleus. *Journal of Neuroscience, 14,* 3588–3602.

Dubin, M. W., Stark, L. A., & Archer, S. M. (1986). A role for action-potential activity in the development of neuronal connections in the kitten retinogeniculate pathway. *Journal of Neuroscience, 6,* 1021–1036.

Dudek, S. M., & Bear, M. F. (1993). Bidirectional long-term modification of synaptic effectiveness in adult and immature hippocampus. *Journal of Neuroscience, 13,* 2910–2918.

Engert, F., & Bonhoeffer, T. (1997). Synapse specificity of long-term potentiation breaks down at short distances. *Nature, 388,* 279–284.

Erzurumlu, R. S., & Guido W. (1996). Cellular mechanisms underlying the formation of orderly connections in developing sensory pathways. *Progress in Brain Research, 108*, 287–301.

Ghosh, A., & Greenberg, M. E. (1995). Calcium signaling in neurons: Molecular mechanisms and cellular consequences. *Science, 268*, 239–247.

Goodman, C. S., & Shatz, C. J. (1993). Developmental mechanisms that generate precise patterns of neuronal connectivity. *Cell (Suppl.), 72*, 77–98.

Guido, W., Lo, F. S., & Erzurumlu, R. S. (2001). Synaptic plasticity in the trigeminal principal nucleus during the period of barrelette formation and consolidation. *Developmental Brain Research, 132*, 97–102.

Guido, W., Tumosa, N., & Spear, P. D. (1989). Binocular interactions in the cat's dorsal lateral geniculate nucleus. I. Spatial-frequency analysis of responses of X, Y, and W cells to nondominant-eye stimulation. *Journal of Neurophysiology, 62*, 526–543.

Hebb, D. O. (1949). *The organization of behavior.* New York: Wiley.

Hermann, K., & Shatz, C. J. (1995). Blockade of action potential activity alters the initial arborization of thalamic axons within cortical layer IV. *Proceedings of the National Academy of Sciences (USA), 92*, 11244–11248.

Jeffery, G. (1984). Retinal ganglion cell death and terminal field retraction in the developing rodent visual system. *Developmental Brain Research, 13*, 81–96.

Kirkwood, A., & Bear, M. F. (1994a). Hebbian synapses in visual cortex. *Journal of Neuroscience, 14*, 1634–1645.

Kirkwood, A., & Bear, M. F. (1994b). Homosynaptic long-term depression in the visual cortex. *Journal of Neuroscience, 14*, 3404–3412.

Kirkwood, A., Dudek, S. M., Aizenman, C. D., & Bear, M. F. (1993). Common forms of synaptic plasticity in the hippocampus and neocortex in vitro. *Science, 260*, 1518–1521.

Liets, L. C., & Chalupa, L. M. (2001). Glutamate-mediated responses in developing retinal ganglion cells. *Progress in Brain Research, 134*, 1–16.

Lindström, S. (1982). Synaptic organization of inhibitory pathways to principal cells in the lateral geniculate nucleus of the cat. *Brain Research, 234*, 447–453.

Lo, F. S., & Mize, R. R. (2000). Synaptic regulation of L-type Ca^{2+} channel activity and long-term depression during refinement of the retinocollicular pathway in developing rodent superior colliculus. *Journal of Neuroscience, 20*, 1–6.

Lo, F. S., Ziburkus, J., & Guido, (2002). W. Synaptic mechanisms regulating the activation of a Ca^{2+}-mediated plateau potential in developing relay cells of the lateral geniculate nucleus. *Journal of Neurophysiology, 87*, 1175–1185.

Lund, R. D., Lund, J. S., & Wise, R. P. (1978). The organization of the retinal projection to the dorsal lateral geniculate nucleus in pigmented and albino rats. *Journal of Comparative Neurology, 158*, 383–404.

Maffei, L., & Galli-Resta, L. (1990). Correlation in the discharges of neighboring rat retinal ganglion cells during prenatal life. *Proceedings of the National Academy of Sciences (USA), 87*, 2861–2864.

Magee, J. C., & Johnston, D. (1997). A synaptically controlled, associative signal for Hebbian plasticity in hippocampal neurons. *Science, 275*, 205–213.

Malenka, R. C., & Siegelbaum, S. A. (2001). Synaptic plasticity: Diverse targets and mechanisms for regulating synaptic efficacy. In W. M. Cowan, T. C. Sudof, & C. F. Stevens (Eds.), *Synapses* (pp. 393–453). Baltimore, MD: Johns Hopkins University Press.

Mastronarde, D. N. (1987). Two classes of single-input X cells in cat lateral geniculate nucleus. II. Retinal inputs and the generation of receptive field properties. *Journal of Neurophysiology, 57*, 381–413.

Miester, M., Wong R. O. L., Baylor, D. A., & Shatz, C. J. (1991). Synchronous bursts of action potentials in ganglion cells of the developing mammalian retina. *Science, 252*, 939–943.

Mooney, R., Penn, A. A., Gallego, R., & Shatz, C. J. (1996). Thalamic relay of spontaneous retinal activity prior to vision. *Neuron, 17*, 863–874.

Munsch, T., Budde, T., & Pape, H. C. (1997). Voltage-activated intracellular calcium transients in thalamic relay cells and interneurons. *Neuroreport, 8*, 2411–2418.

Parnavelas, J. G., Mounty, E. J., Bradford, R., & Lieberman, A. R. (1977). The postnatal development of neurons in the dorsal lateral geniculate nucleus of the rat: A golgi study. *Journal of Comparative Neurology, 171*, 481–500.

Penn, A. A., Riquelme, M. B., Feller, M. B., & Shatz, C. J. (1998). Competition in retinogeniculate patterning driven by spontaneous activity. *Science, 279*, 2108–2112.

Ramoa, A. S., & McCormick, D. A. (1994). Enhanced activation of NMDA receptor responses at the immature retinogeniculate synapse. *Journal of Neuroscience, 14*, 2098–2105.

Ramoa, A. S., & Prusky, G. (1997). Retinal activity regulates developmental switches in functional properties and ifenprodil sensitivity of NMDA receptors in the lateral geniculate nucleus. *Developmental Brain Research, 101,* 165–176.

Reese, B. E. (1988). Hidden lamination in the dorsal lateral geniculate nucleus: The functional organization of this thalamic region in rat. *Brain Research Review, 13,* 119–137.

Reese, B. E., & Cowey, A. (1983). Projection lines and the ipsilateral retino-geniculate pathway in the hooded rat. *Neuroscience, 10,* 1233–1247.

Reese, B. E., & Jeffrey, G. (1983). Crossed and uncrossed visual topography in dorsal lateral geniculate nucleus of the pigmented rat. *Journal of Neurophysiology, 49,* 878–885.

Scharfman, H. E., Lu, S. M., Guido, W., Adams, P. R., & Sherman, S. M. (1990). N-Methyl-D-aspartate (NMDA) receptors contribute to excitatory postsynaptic potentials of cat lateral geniculate neurons recorded in thalamic slices. *Proceedings of the National Academy of Sciences (USA), 87,* 4548–4552.

Schroeder, C. E., Tenke, C. E., Arezzo, J. C., & Vaughan, H. G. (1990). Binocularity in the lateral geniculate nucleus of the alert macaque. *Brain Research, 52,* 303–310.

Schuman, E. M., & Madison, D. V. (1994). Locally distributed synaptic potentiation in the hippocampus. *Science, 263,* 532–536.

Sefton, A. J., & Dreher, B. (1995). Visual system. In G. Paxinos (Ed.), *Rat nervous system* (pp. 833–898). London: Academic Press.

Shatz, C. J. (1990). Impulse activity and the patterning of connections during CNS development. *Neuron, 5,* 745–756.

Shatz, C. J. (1996). Emergence of order in visual system development. *Proceedings of the National Academy of Sciences (USA), 93,* 602–608.

Shatz, C. J., & Stryker, M. P. (1988). Prenatal tetrodotoxin infusion blocks segregation of retinogeniculate afferents. *Science, 242,* 87–89.

Sherman, S. M., & Guillery, R. (1996). The functional organization of thalamocortical relays. *Journal of Neurophysiology, 76,* 1367–1395.

Skailora, I., Scoobey, R. P., & Chalupa, L. M. (1993). Prenatal development of excitability in cat retinal ganglion cells: Action potentials and sodium currents. *Journal of Neuroscience, 13,* 313–323.

Sretavan, D. W., Shatz, C. J., & Stryker, M. P. (1988). Modification of retinal ganglion cell axon morphology by prenatal infusion of tetrodotoxin. *Nature, 336,* 468–471.

Stent, G. S. (1973). A physiological mechanism for Hebb's postulate of learning. *Proceedings of the National Academy of Sciences (USA), 70,* 997–1001.

Tavazoie, S. F., & Reid, R. C. (2000). Diverse receptive fields in the lateral geniculate nucleus during thalamocortical development. *Nature Neuroscience, 3,* 606–616.

Ursey, W. M., Reppas, J. B., & Reid, C. R. (1999). Specificity and strength of retinogeniculate connections. *Journal of Neurophysiology, 82,* 3527–3540.

Wang, G. Y., Ratto, G. M., Bisti, S., & Chalupa, L. M. (1997). Functional development of intrinsic properties in ganglion cells of the mammalian retina. *Journal of Neurophysiology, 78,* 2895–2903.

Webster, M. J., & Rowe, M. H. (1984). Morphology of identified relay cells and interneurons in the dorsal lateral geniculate nucleus of the rat. *Experimental Brain Research, 56,* 468–474.

Weliky, M., & Katz, L. C. (1999). Correlational structure of spontaneous neuronal activity in the developing lateral geniculate nucleus in vivo. *Science, 285,* 599–604.

Wong, R. O. L. (1999). Retinal waves and visual system development. *Annual Review of Neuroscience, 22,* 29–47.

Wong, R. O. L., Miester, M., & Shatz, C. J. (1993). Transient period of correlated bursting activity during the development of the mammalian retina. *Neuron, 11,* 923–938.

Wong, R. O. L., & Oakley, D. M. (1996). Changing patterns of spontaneous bursting activity of on and off retinal ganglion cells during development. *Neuron, 16,* 1087–1095.

Wilson, J. R., Friedlander, M. J., & Sherman, S. M. (1984). Fine structural morphology of identified X- and Y-cells in the cat's lateral geniculate nucleus. *Proceedings of the Royal Society London, Biological Sciences, 221,* 441–486.

Winder, D. G., & Sweatt, D. J. (2001). Roles of serin/threonine phosphatases in hippocampal synaptic plasticity. *Nature Reviews, 2,* 461–474.

6

The Role of Auditory Physiologic Measures in Understanding Human Cortical Function

Linda J. Hood, Ph.D., and Charles I. Berlin, Ph.D.
Kresge Hearing Research Laboratory
Louisiana State University Health Sciences Center
New Orleans, LA

Physiologic responses, including otoacoustic emissions, auditory evoked potentials, and efferent auditory reflexes, provide insight into function of the auditory pathways from the cochlea to the cortex. These objective physiologic measures provide information about auditory pathway integrity, neural synchrony, and central auditory system function and can be used to indirectly estimate auditory sensitivity. Although many of these tests do not truly measure the "moment" of hearing, they are useful in determining the mechanical and neural integrity of the auditory system, which are critical factors in normal hearing. Objective measures show high test sensitivity to underlying neural abnormalities and are advantageous when evaluating young patients and those patients who cannot provide reliable responses on behavioral auditory tasks.

Physiologic responses can be obtained in humans from the cochlea, where otoacoustic emissions (OAEs) are associated with outer hair cell function; from the cochlea, VIIIth nerve, and brain stem pathways via electrocochleography and the auditory brain stem response (ABR); and from the thalamo-cortical pathways, primary and association cortical areas with the middle latency response (MLR), and cortical auditory responses (N1–P2, P300, and mismatch negativity or MMN; see Table 6-1). Efferent function at the level of the peripheral nerve and lower brain stem pathways can be viewed through two acoustic reflexes: the middle-ear muscle reflex (MEMR) and the olivocochlear reflex (OCR). These responses are used to identify the presence of neural pathway disorders resulting from space-occupying lesions as well as more generalized "processing" disorders. The literature on these topics is vast. The following discussion focuses on some underlying principles, characteristics, and applications of physiologic responses and presents two contrasting auditory neural disorders to demonstrate the value of physiologic methods in understanding auditory function and in clinical differential diagnosis.

PRINCIPLES THAT CAN BE APPLIED TO FUNCTIONAL EVALUATION OF THE AUDITORY NERVOUS SYSTEM

Several characteristics of the auditory nervous system exist and are important in evaluating function, interpreting results, and implementing management programs.

Neuromaturation of the Auditory Nervous System

Neural responses recorded even from peripheral portions of the auditory neural pathways continue to develop after birth, and some responses recorded from the cortex continue to mature to age

Table 6-1 Summary of Physiologic Measures of Auditory Function Used in Humans

Cochlear	Afferent Neural	Efferent Neural
Otoacoustic emissions (OAE)	Auditory brainstem response (ABR)	Middle-ear muscle reflex (MEMR)
Cochlear microphonics (CM)	Middle latency response (MLR)	Olivocochlear reflex (OCR)
Summating potential (SP)	Vertex or late response (N1–P2) P300 Mismatch negativity (MMN)	

10 years and beyond. For example, the auditory brain stem response shows decreases in latency over the first 12 to 18 months of age (Starr, Amlie, Martin, & Sanders, 1977), whereas cortical auditory evoked potentials become adultlike in the late teens (e.g., Albrecht, Suchodoletz, & Uwer, 2000; Ponton, Don, Eggermont, Waring, & Masuda, 1996).

Processing at the Peripheral Level

The auditory sensory organ, the cochlea, is composed of inner and outer hair cells that serve very different functions. The main sensory receptors within the cochlea are the inner hair cells that have the majority of the afferent connections to the cochlear branch of the VIIIth cranial nerve. The cochlear outer hair cell system is related to an active process (cochlear amplifier) that is thought to enhance auditory sensitivity and sharpen frequency analysis. The presence of this active process supports observations that frequency tuning and much processing of signals occur in the periphery. The outer hair cells are primarily connected to efferent neural fibers comprising the olivocochlear pathways. Modulation of outer hair cell function via the efferent olivocochlear system may contribute to the ability to process speech in background noise (e.g., Liberman & Guinan, 1998). Measurement of cochlear or otoacoustic emissions, discussed later in this chapter, provides information about outer hair cell system function and may help distinguish peripheral from central disorders. In addition to these acoustic responses, cochlear microphonics and summating potentials are electrical responses from the cochlea recorded via electrocochleography and are used to characterize cochlear function.

Tonotopic Organization

Frequency specificity and tuning in the auditory system begin at the level of the cochlea and are preserved as signals travel to the cortex.

Primary Representation of Stimuli via Contralateral Pathways

The primary neuroanatomical pathway from the ear to the cortex takes a contralateral route with the first decussation occurring at the level of the cochlear nucleus to the contralateral pathways via the trapezoid body. Although this pattern is well known, knowledge of specific generators of certain responses and the relation between performance and sites of dysfunction remain unclear. Consideration of contralateral pathways and crossover of neural pathways at cortical and subcortical levels are important in relating peripheral deficits and performance on auditory processing tests.

Cortical Asymmetries Correlated With Speech-Language Function

Histological and radiological methods demonstrate anatomical asymmetries in the temporal lobes of human brains. The superior surface of the temporal lobe, presumed important for auditory function, is anatomically larger on the left in more brains than the right, and the planum temporale is longer on the left than right in the majority of human subjects (Geschwind, 1978; Geschwind & Levitsky, 1968), more so in males than females (Kulynych, Vlader, Jones, & Weinberger, 1994). Such asymmetries are present in infants and children (Seidenwurm, Bird, Enzmann, & Marshall, 1985; Wada, Clark, & Hamm, 1975; Witelson, 1977). These anatomical asymmetries relate to functional differences between the right and left hemispheres and, in particular, to specialization for speech and language in the left hemisphere (Kimura, 1961; Studdert-Kennedy & Shankweiler, 1970). Newer techniques, such as positron emission tomography, functional magnetic resonance imaging (MRI), or fMRI, and magnetic source imaging enhance the ability to study hemispheric asymmetries and relationships between structural and functional differences (e.g., Belin et al., 1998; Penhune, Zattore, MacDonald, & Evans, 1996; Syzmanski et al., 2001).

Neural Plasticity

Although conventional wisdom might suggest that the nervous system in humans, once fully developed, could not undergo either self-repair or further arborization, clinical observations show that normal humans continue to learn new skills well into their seventies. Reports of patients who had undergone total hemispherectomy and continued to learn new tasks support the reorganization of brain function around remaining strengths. The remarkable recovery of hemispherectomized children was ascribed to the plasticity of their "young brains" and the still incomplete nature of their development, which could then be recruited to compensate for the hemispherectomy. Thus, evidence supports reorganization of the nervous system, or neural plasticity, throughout life as demonstrated through successes in postinjury recovery and specific skill training programs.

AUDITORY PHYSIOLOGIC RESPONSES FROM THE COCHLEA, VIIIth NERVE, AND BRAIN STEM PATHWAYS

Physiologic responses are electric and acoustic in nature. Acoustic responses from the cochlear are measurable as otoacoustic emissions. Electrical responses to auditory stimuli can be recorded from the cochlea to the cortex.

Otoacoustic Emissions

In 1978, Kemp published his now landmark paper outlining the existence of *otoacoustic emissions,* also referred to as cochlear echoes or cochlear emissions (Kemp, 1978). OAEs are low-amplitude acoustic signals that are emitted from the ear and are associated with normally functioning outer hair cells of the cochlea. OAEs do not provide information about function of the cochlear inner hair cells, the primary sensory connection to the VIIIth nerve. Transient-evoked OAEs and distortion product OAEs are the most common OAE measures used clinically, and responses are expected in individuals with normal middle-ear function whose hearing threshold sensitivity is better than 30–40 dB hearing level (HL). OAEs are widely used as a hearing screening test for newborns and infants and as a component of the overall clinical battery of hearing tests used to assess peripheral versus central function in patients of all ages. Coupling OAE measurement with a suppressor stimulus allows assessment of the olivocochlear reflex, as discussed below. Otoacoustic emissions, when used in conjunction with auditory evoked potentials, are particularly helpful in distinguishing disorders (such as in patients with auditory neuropathy/dys-synchrony) that selectively affect the sensorineural pathway while leaving outer hair cell function intact.

Auditory Brain Stem Response

The auditory brain stem response is a robust measure of onset-sensitive single units of the VIIIth nerve and brain stem pathways through the level of the lateral lemniscus. The ABR is present at 26 to 28 weeks gestational age and reaches maturity by 12 to 18 months of age in normal-term infants. The ABR is sensitive to the presence of space-occupying lesions greater than 1 cm affecting the VIIIth nerve, brain stem, or both (Starr & Achor, 1975), whereas imaging studies are often used to identify and confirm small lesions and multiple sclerosis. The ABR is generally absent in patients with auditory nerve dys-synchrony (auditory neuropathy; Starr, Picton, Sininger, Hood, & Berlin, 1996) but is generally normal in children with auditory processing disorders at thalamic and higher levels in the auditory system (Hood, Berlin, & Allen, 1994). Thus, a normal ABR does not rule out deficits that may interfere with normal development of speech and language. Further information about the ABR can be found in Hood (1998) and Hall (1992). Although the ABR is clearly associated with subcortical activity, it is often used as part of a test battery to determine involvement of eighth nerve and lower brain stem pathways.

AUDITORY PHYSIOLOGIC RESPONSES ASSOCIATED WITH CORTICAL PATHWAYS

Middle latency responses (MLR) and certain "late" responses (e.g., N1–P2) represent onset-sensitive responses from the cortical auditory pathways. Middle latency and cortical responses display abnormalities in patients with space-occupying lesions as well as functional abnormalities. These responses are affected by age and subject state (e.g., the influence of sleep and sedation), and the identification of abnormalities may require specialized recording methods. In-depth discussion of the middle latency and cortical responses can be found in Kraus and McGee (1992) and McPherson (1996).

Auditory Middle Latency Response (MLR)

The MLR was among the first auditory evoked potentials recorded from the human scalp (Geisler, Frishkopf, & Rosenblith, 1958). It consists of activity occurring between about 8 and 80 msec poststimulus onset and a series of vertex-positive peaks that are labeled Po, Pa, and Pb and vertex-negative peaks labeled Na and Nb (see Figure 6-1). There are two primary vertex-positive components noted as Wave Pa at approximately 30 msec poststimulation

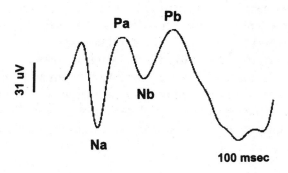

Figure 6-1. Normal middle latency response.

and Wave Pb at 50–55 msec. The earliest component (Po) is believed to primarily represent brain stem and myogenic activity, whereas the Pa and Pb components are neural in origin (Harker, Hosick, Voots, & Mendel, 1977; Kileny, 1983). Although the MLR generators have not been conclusively isolated, centers in the thalamus (medial geniculate) and primary cortical projections in auditory areas are likely candidates (Erwin & Buchwald, 1986; Kraus, McGee, & Comperatore, 1990; Ozdamar & Kraus, 1983; Picton, Hillyard, Krausz, & Galambos, 1974). There are distinct primary and nonprimary pathways with components that are differentially affected by arousal state and have different maturational time courses (McGee & Kraus, 1996). MLRs may be recorded in young children but may not reach normal values until 8 to 10 years of age. The MLR is sensitive to handedness, with left-handed listeners generally showing longer Wave Pb latencies than right-handed listeners (Hood, Martin, & Berlin, 1990).

Evaluation of Disorders of the Central Auditory Pathways With MLR

The MLR has proven useful in the evaluation of central auditory disorders. Patients with bilateral temporal lobe lesions generally show abnormal MLRs (Hood et al., 1994; Ozdamar, Kraus, & Curry, 1982;), although normal MLRs have also been reported (Parving, Salomon, Elberling, Larsen, & Lassen, 1980). Unilateral temporal lobe lesions may be missed if only a vertex electrode is used. Kraus, Ozdamar, Hier, and Stein (1982) describe the use of electrodes over each temporal lobe as well and show that MLR amplitude decreases for recordings from the electrode montage ipsilateral to the lesion. Higher incidences of abnormal MLRs have also been reported in language-impaired children than in children with normal language development. When evaluating the MLR, the response is examined for replicability, presence or absence of the response, symmetry of responses resulting from stimulation of each ear, symmetry of recordings obtained over each hemisphere, and whether latency of the major peaks falls within the expected time regions.

Late Potentials: N1–P2

Cortical responses include those obtained to like stimuli either in quiet or in competing message situations (e.g., N1–P2 response) as well as those involving discrimination between different stimuli where a response is required (e.g., P300) or where no response is necessary (e.g., mismatch negativity). As a historical note, cortical responses were recorded long before the ABR and MLR. In 1939, Pauline Davis reported the recording of an evoked potential elicited from the awake human brain in response to auditory stimuli; in that same year, Hallowell Davis recorded an auditory evoked potential from the sleeping brain. These responses were the N1–P2 response, also referred to as the vertex or "V" potential, because the amplitude is greatest from an electrode placed at the vertex (Figure 6-2). Putative generators of the N1–P2 response include supratemporal auditory cortex and nonspecific polysensory system (McPherson, 1996)

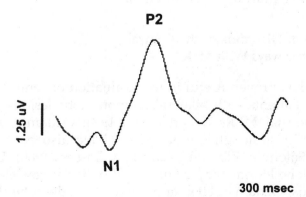

Figure 6-2. Normal N1–P2 cortical response to tones.

Event-Related Potentials (P300 and Mismatch Negativity)

Cortical potentials such as the P300 response and mismatch negativity (MMN) are "event-related potentials" that occur when the brain makes a decision about whether one stimulus differs from another. For these responses, two different stimuli are presented in an "odd-ball" paradigm in which one stimulus is presented frequently (e.g., 80% of the stimuli) and the other stimulus is presented more rarely (e.g., 20% of the time). When recording the P300 response, the patient is asked to keep track only of the rare stimuli that result in generation of a neural potential occurring in the 300-msec poststimulus latency range (Figure 6-3). P300 is a cognitive response dependent on focusing of attention and subtle cognitive processes. Davis (1964) provided one of the earliest descriptions of the effects of attention and discrimination of acoustic signals on auditory evoked potentials. Hillyard, Hink, Schwent, and Picton (1973) describe another method of demonstrating attention to selected stimuli. Thus, the P300 can be recorded using speech stimuli of various types (discrimination, semantic distinctions, etc.). It is also possible to probe psychophysical function (discrimination of two tones, etc.).

The MMN uses a similar paradigm; in this case, however, no response is required from the patient. The MMN is a neural response to minimal changes in acoustic stimuli that is objective and passively elicited. It is sensitive to processing within auditory cortex; can be used to probe frequency, intensity, and temporal discrimination; and has implications for speech processing. The MMN can be recorded without participation of the patient, other than remaining quiet, making it particularly useful in evaluating

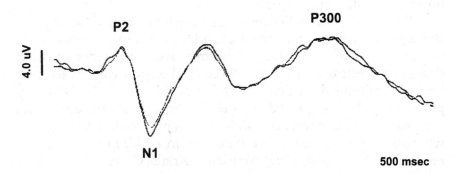

Figure 6-3. Normal P300 response to tones.

infants and young children. Unlike other cortical auditory potentials, the MMN is quite stable developmentally and can be obtained from even preterm infants (Cheour-Lutanen et al., 1996). Amplitude shows little change across age, and latency reaches adultlike values by school-age years. The MMN appears to be a promising technique in understanding various auditory perception abilities (e.g., Kraus et al., 1995; Kraus, McGee, & Koch, 1998). Phoneme discrimination has been demonstrated with the MMN in children and adults and in relation to foreign language learning and foreign versus native language processing (Kraus et al., 1995; Naatanen et al., 1997; Winkler et al., 1999). The MMN also has been used to demonstrate phoneme discrimination ability in infants as young as 30 to 34 weeks conceptional age (Cheour et al., 1996) and to study development of language specific discrimination abilities (Cheour et al., 1998).

Applications of Cortical Potentials

Cortical responses are promising techniques in enhancing understanding of auditory perception abilities in children and adults, assessing the effectiveness of cochlear implants, monitoring the effectiveness of intervention programs, and studying the effects of aging on the auditory system (Cheour, Leppanen, & Kraus, 2000; Jerger, Alford, Lew, Rivera, & Chmiel, 1995; Kraus et al., 1995; Tonnquist-Uhlen, 1996). It is possible to probe processing of fine acoustic differences whose discrimination is fundamental to speech perception and characterize processes involved in encoding speech. Such auditory processing abilities are fundamental to language acquisition, because many children with auditory processing disorders, learning problems, or both require larger than normal acoustic differences.

The MMN and P300 responses have been used to explore changes in auditory function as a result of some intervention, consistent with neural plasticity. Children and adults demonstrate changes in vertex N1–P2 and P300 cortical responses between pre- and posttraining conditions. In children identified with auditory processing difficulties, P300 latency showed significant shifts towards normal control values following auditory training, whereas responses remained abnormal in children who did not receive training (Jirsa, 1992). Tremblay, Kraus, Carrell, and McGee (1997) report MMN results obtained in adults before and after listening training. English-speaking adults who were trained on a non-English sound generated larger MMN responses after training than control subjects who did not receive training. They also showed transfer of training to another sound that was not included in the training sessions. Such studies demonstrate that neurophysiologic processes underlying perceptual learning can be altered through auditory training.

Cortical responses that probe discrimination ability also have been studied in cochlear implant patients. P300 responses tend to be stronger in successful cochlear implant users and show promise in monitoring progress and discrimination ability in implant patients (Kileny, 1991). Significant correlations between speech recognition and cognitive evoked potential latencies support the clinical use of cognitive evoked potentials in children with cochlear implants (Kileny, Boerst, & Zwolan, 1997).

Neuropathological Findings of Cortical Potentials

Middle latency and cortical responses display abnormalities in patients with disorders at suprathalamic/supracollicular levels of the auditory system. Abnormal MLRs are reported in individuals with unilateral and bilateral lesions of the temporal lobes (Kileny, Paccioretti, & Wilson, 1987; Kraus et al., 1982; Ozdamar et al., 1982). Abnormal cortical responses are associated with a number of neurological disorders including Huntington disease, Parkinson's disease, HIV, Alzheimer's disease, schizophrenia, autism, and dementia. MLRs and cortical potentials are affected by sleep and sedation, are susceptible to muscle activity, and have longer neuromaturational time courses than the ABR. Although these responses may be more difficult to record reliably in young children, they hold significant value in learning about central auditory processing in normal and abnormal systems. In-depth discussions of the middle latency and cortical responses can be found in Kraus and McGee (1992) and McPherson (1996).

EFFERENT AUDITORY REFLEXES

There are two efferent reflexes of the auditory system that can be assessed in humans: the middle-ear muscle reflex and the olivo-cochlear reflex. Both of these responses reflect activity of pathways from the auditory branch of the vestibulocochlear nerve and the lower brain stem pathways. Patients with auditory nerve or lower brain stem disorders generally show abnormal MEMR and OCR responses, whereas patients with cortical disorders and intact subcortical pathways should show normal responses to these efferent reflexes.

Middle-Ear Muscle Reflex

The MEMR, which occurs in response to high-intensity acoustic stimuli, results in measurable contraction of the stapedius muscle. This response depends on an intact reflex arc involving the middle-ear system, afferent VIIIth cranial nerve and caudal brain stem auditory pathways, and efferent activation of the VIIth (facial) nerve. Stimulation of one ear with high-intensity stimuli normally results in bilateral contraction of the stapedius muscles, provided that the middle ears, as well as pathways of the VIIth and VIIIth cranial nerves and lower brain stem tracts through the superior olivary complex, are intact. The MEMR has proven to be a robust measure of the integrity of neural pathways in patients with space-occupying lesions of the VIIIth nerve and in patients with auditory neuropathy. Although a very sensitive measure, the middle-ear muscle reflexes are compromised by conductive (middle-ear) disorders, Bell's palsy, cochlear hearing losses greater than moderate in degree, and neural abnormalities affecting the VIIth or VIIIth nerves or brain stem pathways. Comparing middle-ear muscle reflexes obtained with both ipsilateral and contralateral stimulation provides insight into the nature and possible area of a problem. For example, the presence of ipsilateral reflexes and absence of contralateral reflexes is pathognomic for caudal brain stem dysfunction. Because of the effectiveness of MEMR measurement and the brief amount of time necessary to obtain information, its use as a routine clinical measure in clinical practice is recommended.

The Olivocochlear Reflex and Efferent Suppression of Otoacoustic Emissions

A second efferent reflex in the auditory system, the *olivocochlear reflex*, reflects activity at the level of the caudal brain stem and affects outer hair cell function. The OCR can be measured by *efferent suppression of OAEs*. This response occurs as a result of activation of the medial efferent pathways descending via the olivo-cochlear bundle to the outer hair cells. Efferent OAE suppression, or the OCR, is measured clinically by comparing OAEs obtained with and without introduction of a suppressor stimulus. Efferent suppression can be assessed using continuous noise in the ear contralateral to the OAE stimulus (Berlin, Hood, Wen, et al., 1993; Collet et al., 1990; Ryan, Kemp, & Hinchcliffe, 1991) or by presenting a suppressor stimulus contralaterally, ipsilaterally, or binaurally using a forward masking paradigm (Berlin, Hood, Hurley, Wen, & Kemp, 1995). In a forward masking paradigm, the suppressor stimulus (which may be thought of as the "masker" in forward masking terminology) precedes the OAE evoking stimulus in time so as to avoid interactions between two stimuli presented simultaneously through the same earphone. Efferent suppression is characterized by amplitude decreases and phase shifts in the OAEs (Berlin, Hood, Wen, et al., 1993; Collet et al., 1990; Ryan et al., 1991).

The ability to measure the OCR depends on the presence of OAEs, which is expected in individuals with peripheral hearing sensitivity better than 30 to 40 dB HL, and normal middle-ear function. Efferent suppression is not present at birth in all infants (Goforth, Hood, & Berlin, 1997; Goforth-Barter et al., 2000; Morlet, Collet, Salle, & Morgon, 1993; Morlet et al., 1999; Ryan & Piron, 1994) and shows aging effects particularly under binaural suppression conditions (Castor, Veuillet, Morgon, & Collet, 1994; Hood, Hurley, Goforth, Bordelon, & Berlin, 1997). Efferent suppression of OAEs is abnormal in patients with vestibular nerve section (Williams, Brookes, & Prasher, 1994), in patients with auditory neuropathy/auditory dys-synchrony (Berlin, Hood, Cecola, Jackson, & Szabo, 1993), and in many patients with tumors affecting the VIIIth nerve (Maurer, Beck, Mann, & Minter, 1992).

Analysis of Efferent Suppression of Transient OAEs

A consistent observation throughout these studies and those of others is the occurrence of maximal suppression in the 8- to 18-msec time period after the onset of the click (e.g., Berlin, Hood, Wen, et al., 1993; Collet et al., 1990). Because suppression effects are greater in some time or frequency regions than in others, a single value cannot adequately represent the maximal effects or define time regions containing the greatest amount of suppression. In fact, an overall aggregate number will underestimate the suppression effect in many subjects. To obtain more detailed analysis, a method was developed (Kresge EchoMaster Program) to analyze suppression of emissions in greater detail (Wen, Berlin, Hood, Jackson, & Hurley, 1993). The EchoMaster program provides comparisons of (a) two individual emissions, (b) the means of two groups of emissions with up to 60 emissions in each group, and (c) an individual emission with its estimated background noise. An example of an EchoMaster comparison of two emissions across time and frequency is shown in Figure 6-4.

Typically, root-mean-square amplitude differences between the "with" and "without" noise conditions are evaluated. Amplitude effects can be plotted in 1-, 2-, or 3-msec intervals. When subjects have low-amplitude emissions or if a subject's records are noisy, an estimate of the interrun variability can be

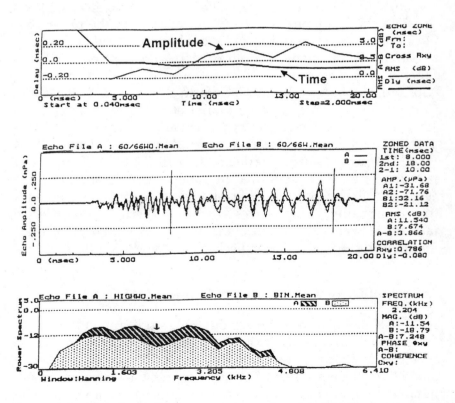

Figure 6-4. Analysis of OAE suppression using the EchoMaster program. Shown are comparisons between with and without suppressor stimulus across time (top and middle panels) and frequency (bottom panel). (Adapted from Figures 5-1 and 5-5 in Hood, Berlin, Goforth-Barter, Bordelon, & Wen, 1999.)

obtained. This estimate is useful in assuring that differences between conditions with and without suppressor noise truly are an effect of the noise and are not simply due to run-to-run variability. This procedure is especially useful in infants where noise levels may be higher than usual and in individuals with low-amplitude OAEs. Efferent suppression effects also can be quantified by frequency. Spectral analysis is useful in understanding the characteristics of efferent suppression and how it may vary among subject groups. For example, it has been observed that although infant emissions often show higher frequency content, the frequency characteristics of suppression are quite similar to those of adults (Goforth et al., 1997).

EVALUATING AUDITORY PROCESSING

Although the incidence of auditory processing disorders of the peripheral and central nervous systems is lower than the more peripheral (middle-ear and cochlear) hearing disorders, these disorders have significant effects on speech perception and language learning. Individuals with deficits of the auditory neural pathways often demonstrate normal peripheral hearing and normal results on measures of the auditory system that involve tonal or speech stimuli presented only to one ear and without competition. Routine measures of pure tone thresholds and speech recognition in quiet are generally insensitive to auditory processing deficits. They are, however, unable to successfully use more complex auditory stimuli, particularly in adverse listening conditions. Measures that are sensitive to auditory processing disorders introduce a temporally competing signal in either the same ear (monotic) or opposite ear (dichotic), use binaural presentation to test interaction of signals, or involve some type of distortion that alters the frequency, intensity, or temporal characteristics of signals.

Because ability to process signals in the central auditory system is influenced by peripheral hearing loss, proper interpretation of test results is not possible without knowledge of peripheral hearing sensitivity. Advantages of physiological over behavioral measures include a lack of dependence on attention, motivation, reading ability, educational background, linguistic function, and fatigability. Furthermore, many behavioral tests exhibit considerable inherent variability, particularly when used with younger age groups.

A broad range of auditory processing problems exist, and the presenting characteristics (Table 6-2) are often similar. Two types of auditory processing disorders that affect neural processing in different portions of the auditory pathways, however, can be distinguished. They are distinct both in the sites of the neural disorder and in the type of management that is successful. In Table 6-3, typical findings in patients with auditory neuropathy/dys-synchrony (e.g., Berlin, Hood, Cecola, et al., 1993; Berlin, Hood, Morlet, & Keats, 2001; Starr et al., 1996) are compared with those in patients with auditory processing disorders localizable the cortical level (e.g., Hood et al., 1994).

Table 6-2 Alerting Signs and Symptoms Associated With Auditory Processing Disorders

Normal audiogram but speech audiometric loss
Teacher reports that child does not always seem to hear
Misses assignments, says never got them
Reduced auditory attention span
Makes mistakes in sound localization
Gets confused when several people are talking
More problems with one ear than the other

Table 6-3 Test Results in Auditory Neuropathy/Dys-synchrony and Cortical Deafness

Measure	Auditory Neuropathy/ Auditory Dys-synchrony	Cortical Deafness
Otoacoustic emissions	Normal	Normal
Cochlear microphonics	Present	Present
Auditory brain stem response	Absent	Normal
Middle latency response	Abnormal	Abnormal
Late responses	Normal or abnormal	Abnormal
Middle-ear muscle reflex	Absent	Normal
Olivocochlear reflex	Absent	Normal

AUDITORY NEUROPATHY/DYS-SYNCHRONY: AN AUDITORY PROCESSING PROBLEM DUE TO POOR NEURAL SYNCHRONY OR A PERIPHERAL NEUROPATHY

Patients ranging in age from infants to adults have been described with a disorder called auditory neuropathy or auditory dys-synchrony (Berlin, Hood, Cecola, et al., 1993; Berlin, Hood, & Rose, 2001; Starr et al., 1996). These patients demonstrate normal outer hair cell function evidenced by the presence of otoacoustic emissions and cochlear microphonics. Abnormal neural responses are reflected by absent ABRs, absent MEMRs, and abnormal efferent reflexes, including MEMRs and efferent suppression of OAEs (Hood & Berlin, 2001). Although there sometimes appears to be an ABR, close examination shows no latency change with decreasing stimulus intensity and response inversion when the polarity of the stimulus is reversed (rarefaction versus condensation clicks), consistent with cochlear microphonics (Berlin et al., 1998). Pure-tone thresholds vary from normal sensitivity to the severe or profound hearing loss range (e.g., Berlin, Hood, Cecola, et al., 1993; Berlin, Hood, Hurley, & Wen, 1994; Gorga, Stelmachowicz, Barlow, & Brookhouser, 1995; Kaga et al., 1996; Starr et al., 1991). Patients generally show no masking level differences, consistent with abnormalities in processing of phase information and a disturbance in timing and neural synchrony (Starr et al., 1991, Zeng, Oba, Garde, Sininger, & Starr, 1999). Speech recognition is quite variable, although generally much poorer than expected and particularly poor in noise. Patients with auditory neuropathy/dys-synchrony show normal computed tomography (CT) and MRI results, which distinguishes them from patients with space-occupying lesions or disorders such as multiple sclerosis.

The classification of auditory neuropathy/dys-synchrony most likely describes several different specific sites of abnormality, all of which result in the clinical observation of normal outer hair cell responses accompanied by poor neural synchrony. Most writers agree with Starr et al. (1991) that this abnormality is a timing disorder that may be axonic, dendritic, or even primarily sensory in nature. The mechanical transduction or other functional characteristics of the inner hair cells could be abnormal, the synaptic juncture between the inner hair cells and the cochlear branch of the vestibulocochlear (VIIIth) nerve could be affected, or the axons or cell bodies of the VIIIth nerve itself could be the site. Uneven conduction velocities, especially in cases in which there is demyelization, could underlie the poor synchrony observed. Patients with auditory neuropathy are distinguished from those with space-occupying lesions (such as vestibular schwannoma) because imaging studies in patients with auditory neuropathy are normal. Some patients, both children and adults, have no known etiology and no other identified neurological abnormalities. In other patients, the auditory findings may be associated with other peripheral neuropathies such as hereditary motor sensory neuropathy (Charcot-Marie-Tooth disease). Of particular interest is the number of infants and young children who have been identified with auditory dys-synchrony. Infants with neonatal abnormalities, including prematurity, exchange transfusion, low birth weight, and hyperbilirubinemia, have been reported (Deltenre, Mansbach, Bozet, Clercx, & Hecox, 1997; Stein et al., 1996), and there are cases in which a genetic basis is suspected due to multiple affected family members (Berlin, Hood, Marlet, & Keats, 2001).

The majority of patients with auditory neuropathy/dys-synchrony patients who have been managed with cochlear implants demonstrate good benefit. Some reports advocate the use of hearing for these patients (e.g., Rance et al., 1999). Although hearing aids sometimes improve sensitivity in quiet, management of patients with auditory neuropathy/dys-synchrony by auditory means alone has not led to language development. Some patients benefit from frequency modulation devices, most likely due to improved signal-to-noise ratios that provide a clearer signal to a system that cannot cope with interference. Management for all children with auditory neuropathy/dys-synchrony should include use of some visual system (such as cued speech or sign language) to facilitate development of language and communication skills. Although patients do well with auditory/verbal therapy post-cochlear implant, auditory cues alone are insufficient for language development in these patients.

LOCALIZABLE CORTICAL HEARING DEFICITS

Patients with cortical deafness, also referred to as central auditory deafness, auditory aphasia, or verbal auditory agnosia, present unique evaluation and habilitation challenges (e.g., Goldstein, 1974; Graham, Greenwood, & Lecky, 1980; Jerger, Weikers, Sharbrough,

& Jerger, 1969; Kaga, Shindo, & Tanaka, 1997; Landau, Goldstein, & Kleffner, 1957; Landau & Kleffner, 1957; Michel, Peronnet, & Schott, 1980). Of particular interest is the case reported by Landau and colleagues (1957) of a child who by 6 years of age had not developed speech, despite apparent adequate intelligence. Reactions were observed to low-frequency sounds, but no comprehension of spoken language was apparent. At 8 years, a functional vocabulary of about 175 words was present via reading, speaking, and writing. Following the child's death at age 10 due to cardiac complications, the child's brain was obtained for examination. The brain stem was grossly normal; cortical degeneration of the parietal, temporal, and occipital lobes was observed, however, and the medial geniculate nuclei were severely degenerated. This case demonstrated severe anatomical damage to the primary auditory projection pathways bilaterally and the near complete effect on speech and language development. This patient fit the characteristics of Landau-Kleffner syndrome, or acquired aphasia with convulsive disorder (Landau & Kleffner, 1957), with approximately 200 cases reported in the literature (Klein, Tuchman, & Rapin, 2000).

One patient with cortical deafness has been followed at Kresge Hearing Research Laboratory for more than 20 years (Hood et al., 1994). Following a high fever at about 1 year of age, several misdiagnoses were made over the years that followed including peripheral deafness, learning disability, emotional disturbance, retardation, and autism. When the authors first saw her, she was 5 years old, was unable to follow verbal instructions, and demonstrated speech quality that is characteristic of individuals with profound hearing loss. Peripheral auditory sensitivity was difficult to quantify due to inconsistent responses; thresholds for speech stimuli were in the normal-to-mild hearing loss range. Middle-ear muscle reflexes were normal. Good peripheral hearing sensitivity was confirmed by auditory brain stem responses to low- and high-frequency stimuli where latency-intensity functions showed responses to very faint stimuli for each ear. Thus, peripheral sensitivity was considered normal bilaterally. Middle latency responses were absent bilaterally, which was consistent with bilateral absence of large portions of the temporal lobes shown by CT and later by MRI. Late cortical responses showed the presence of some synchronous activity but with delays in latency and asymmetries in amplitude. The patient's inability to recognize speech stimuli precluded all speech-based behavioral central hearing tests.

Localization testing showed inability to reliably localize any stimuli. As would be expected, this child received little to no benefit from speech therapy or hearing aids. In fact, she rejected hearing aids and communicated primarily by reading and writing until learning sign language. Her language ability remains significantly delayed, and she relies on manual communication.

CONTRASTING PERIPHERAL NEURAL FROM MORE CENTRAL AUDITORY NEURAL DISORDERS

Several useful points are learned by comparing these two types of auditory neural disorders. First, auditory neuropathy/dys-synchrony and more "central" auditory processing disorders are contrasted by the site of the disorder and by the pattern of test results. Second, the use of objective measures of auditory function was critical to understanding the source of both hearing disorders. Third, objective tests such as the ABR and MEMRs do not evaluate and cannot be used to eliminate the possibility of a more central hearing loss. Fourth, it is important to look beyond peripheral auditory areas when communication problems cannot be explained. Fifth, management options also differ in that cochlear implants have been successful in the majority of auditory neuropathy/dys-synchrony patients implanted, whereas cochlear implants are not a management option for more centrally based auditory processing disorders. And finally, identification of problems anywhere in the neural auditory pathways must be followed *immediately* by appropriate management and assurance that the patient has a viable mode of communication.

CONCLUSIONS

Physiological measures of the peripheral and central auditory pathways focus on assessment of the functional integrity of the auditory system and can be used to assess integrity and function from the cochlea to the cortex. They provide sources of information about neural development, noninvasive methods of assessing speech encoding and perception, and objective methods of documenting neural plasticity associated with treatment and training programs. Clinical value is very strong, as demonstrated by the use of patterns of responses in differential diagnosis. Middle-ear measurements, including assessment of ipsilateral and contralateral MEMRs, are included in the basic audiological test battery in many progressive clinical practices. The value of the combination of OAEs and measures of neural function at the level of the VIIIth nerve and brain stem is demonstrated in the clinical assessment of patients with auditory neuropathy/dys-synchrony. Auditory evoked potentials that assess various portions of the auditory system from the brain stem to the cortex are useful in identifying patients with cortical auditory abnormalities.

ACKNOWLEDGMENT

Preparation of this chapter was supported by the National Institute on Deafness and Other Communication Disorders, Oberkotter Foundation, Deafness Research Foundation, National Organization for Hearing Research, and KAM's Fund for Hearing Research.

REFERENCES

Albrecht, R., Suchodoletz, W., & Uwer, R. (2000). The development of auditory evoked dipole source activity from childhood to adulthood. *Clinical Neurophysiology, 111*, 2268–2276.

Belin, P., Zilbovicious, M., Crozier, S., Thivard, L., Fontaine, A., Masure, M. C., et al. (1998). Lateralization of speech and auditory temporal processing. *Journal of Cognitive Neuroscience, 10*, 536–540.

Berlin, C., Hood, L., & Rose, K. (2001). On renaming auditory neuropathy as auditory dys-synchrony: Implications for a clearer understanding of the underlying mechanisms and management options. *Audiology Today, 13*, 15–17.

Berlin, C. I., Bordelon, J., St. John, P., Wilensky, D., Hurley, A., Kluka, E., et al. (1998). Reversing click polarity may uncover auditory neuropathy in infants. *Ear and Hearing, 19*, 37–47.

Berlin, C. I., Hood, L. J., Cecola, R. P., Jackson, D. F., & Szabo, P. (1993). Does type I afferent neuron dysfunction reveal itself through lack of efferent suppression? *Hearing Research, 65*, 40–50.

Berlin, C. I., Hood, L. J., Hurley, A., & Wen, H. (1994). Contralateral suppression of otoacoustic emissions: An index of the function of the medial olivocochlear system. *Otolaryngology—Head Neck Surgery, 100,* 3–21.

Berlin, C. I., Hood, L. J., Hurley, A., Wen, H., & Kemp, D. T. (1995). Bilateral noise suppresses click-evoked otoacoustic emissions more than ipsilateral or contralateral noise. *Hearing Research, 87,* 96–103.

Berlin, C. I., Hood, L. J., Morlet, T., & Keats, B. J. (2001). Managing and renaming auditory neuropathy (AN) as part of a continuum of auditory dys-synchrony (AD). *ARO Abstracts, 24,* 137.

Berlin, C. I., Hood, L. J., Wen, H., Szabo, P., Cecola, R. P., Rigby, P., et al. (1993). Contralateral suppression of non-linear click-evoked otoacoustic emissions in humans. *Hearing Research, 71,* 1–11.

Bocca, E., & Calearo, C. (1963). Central hearing processes. In J. Jerger (Ed.), *Modern developments in audiology* (pp. 337–370). New York: Academic Press.

Castor, X., Veuillet, E., Morgon, A., & Collet, L. (1994). Influence of aging on active cochlear micromechanical properties and on the medial olivocochlear system in humans. *Hearing Research, 77,* 1–8.

Cheour, M., Ceponiene, R., Lehtokoski, A., Luuk, A., Allik, J., Ahlo, K., et al. (1998). Development of language-specific phoneme representations in the infant brain. *Nature Neuroscience, 1,* 351–353.

Cheour, M., Leppanen, P. H. T., & Kraus, N. (2000). Mismatch negativity (MMN) as a tool for investigating auditory discrimination and sensory memory in infants and children. *Clinical Neurophysiology, 111,* 4–16.

Cheour-Lutanen, M., Alho, K., Sainio, K., Rinne, T., Reinikainen, K., Pohjavuori, M., et al. (1996). The ontogenetically earliest discriminative response of the human brain. *Psychophysiology, 33,* 478–481.

Collet, L., Kemp, D. T., Veuillet, E., Duclaux, R., Moulin, A., & Morgon, A. (1990). Effect of contralateral auditory stimuli on active cochlear micro-mechanical properties in human subjects. *Hearing Research, 43,* 251–262.

Davis, H. (1964). Enhancement of evoked cortical potentials in humans related to a task requiring a decision. *Science, 145,* 182–183.

Deltenre, P., Mansbach, A. L., Bozet, C., Clercx, A., & Hecox, K. E. (1997). Auditory neuropathy: A report on three cases with early onsets and major neonatal illnesses. *Electroencephalography and Clinical Neurophysiology, 104,* 17–22.

Erwin, R. J., & Buchwald, J. S. (1986). Midlatency auditory evoked responses: Differential recovery cycle characteristics. *Electroencephalography and Clinical Neurophysiology, 64,* 417–423.

Fernald, A., & Kuhl, P. (1987). Acoustic determinants of infant perception for motherese speech. *Infant Behavior Development, 10,* 279.

Geisler, C. D., Frishkopf, L. S., & Rosenblith, W. A. (1958). Extracranial responses to acoustic clicks in man. *Science, 128,* 1210–1211.

Geschwind, N. (1978). Anatomical asymmetry as the basis for cerebral dominance. *Federal Proceedings, 37,* 2263–2266.

Geschwind, N., & Levitsky, W. (1968). Human brain: Left-right asymmetries in temporal speech region. *Science, 161,* 186–187.

Goforth, L., Hood, L. J., & Berlin, C. I. (1997). Efferent suppression of transient-evoked otoacoustic emissions in human infants. *ARO Abstracts, 20,* 166.

Goforth-Barter, L., Hood, L. J., Li, L., Morlet, T., Reddy, S., & Berlin, C. I. (2000). Update on the development of neonatal auditory efferent function. *ARO Abstracts, 23,* 159.

Goldstein, M. N. (1974). Auditory agnosia for speech ("pure word deafness"). *Brain and Language, 1,* 195–204.

Gorga, M. P., Stelmachowicz, P. G., Barlow, S. M., & Brookhouser, P. E. (1995). Case of recurrent, reversible, sudden sensorineural hearing loss in a child. *Journal of the American Academy of Audiology, 6,* 163–172.

Graham, J., Greenwood, R., & Lecky, B. (1980). Cortical deafness: A case report and review of the literature. *Journal of Neurological Sciences, 48,* 35–49.

Hall, J. W., III. (1992). *Handbook of auditory evoked responses.* Boston: Allyn and Bacon.

Harker, L. A., Hosick, E., Voots, R. J., & Mendel, M. I. (1977). Influence of succinylcholine on middle-component auditory evoked potentials. *Archives of Otolaryngology, 103,* 133–137.

Hillyard, S. A., Hink, R. F., Schwent, V. L., & Picton, T. W. (1973). Electrical signs of selective attention in the human brain. *Science, 182,* 177–180.

Hood, L. J. (1998). *Clinical applications of the auditory brainstem response.* Clifton Park, NY: Delmar Learning.

Hood, L. J., & Berlin, C. I. (2001). Efferent suppression in patients with auditory neuropathy. In Y. S. Sininger & A. Starr (Eds.),

Auditory neuropathy: A new perspective on hearing disorders (pp. 183–202). Clifton Park, NY: Delmar Learning.

Hood, L. J., Berlin, C. I., & Allen, P. (1994). Cortical deafness: A longitudinal study. *Journal of the American Academy of Audiology, 5,* 330–342.

Hood, L. J., Berlin, C. I., Goforth-Barter, L., Bordelon, J., & Wen, H. (1999). Recording and analyzing efferent suppression of transient-evoked otoacoustic emissions. In C. I. Berlin (Ed.), *The efferent auditory system.* Clifton Park, NY: Delmar Learning.

Hood, L. J., Hurley, A. E., Goforth, L., Bordelon, J., & Berlin, C. I. (1997). Aging and efferent suppression of otoacoustic emissions. *ARO Abstracts, 20,* 167.

Hood, L. J., Martin, D. A., & Berlin, C. I. (1990). Auditory evoked potentials differ at 50 milliseconds in right- and left-handed listeners. *Hearing Research, 45,* 115–122.

Jerger, J., Alford, B., Lew, H., Rivera, V., & Chmiel, R. (1995). Dichotic listening, event-related potentials, and interhemispheric transfer in the elderly. *Ear and Hearing, 16,* 482–498.

Jerger, J., Weikers, N. J., Sharbrough, F. W., & Jerger, S. (1969). Bilateral lesions of the temporal lobe: A case study. *Acta Otolaryngologica: Supplement, 258,* 1–57.

Jirsa, R. E. (1992). The clinical utility of the P3 AERP in children with auditory processing disorders. *Journal of Speech and Hearing Research, 35,* 903–912.

Kaga, K., Nakamura, M., Shinogami, M., Tsuzuku, T., Yamada, K., & Shindo, M. (1996). Auditory nerve disease of both ears revealed by auditory brainstem responses, electrocochleography and otoacoustic emissions. *Scandinavian Audiology, 25,* 233–238.

Kaga, K., Shindo, M., & Tanaka, Y. (1997). Central auditory information processing in patients with bilateral auditory cortex lesions. *Acta Oto-Laryngologica (Suppl.), 532,* 77–82.

Kemp, D. T. (1978). Stimulated acoustic emissions from within the human auditory system. *Journal of the Acoustical Society of America, 64,* 1386–1391.

Kileny, P. (1983). Auditory evoked middle latency responses: Current issues. *Seminars in Hearing, 4,* 403–413.

Kileny, P., Paccioretti, D., & Wilson, A. F. (1987). Effects of cortical lesions on middle-latency auditory evoked responses. *Electroencephalography and Clinical Neurophysiology, 66,* 108–120.

Kileny, P. R. (1991). Use of electrophysiologic measures in the management of children with cochlear implants: Brainstem, middle latency, and cognitive (P300) responses. *American Journal of Otology, 12,* 37–42.

Kileny, P. R., Boerst, A., & Zwolan, T. (1997). Cognitive evoked potentials to speech and tonal stimuli in children with implants. *Otolaryngology—Head and Neck Surgery, 117,* 161–169.

Kimura, D. (1961). Cerebral dominance and the perception of verbal stimuli. *Canadian Journal of Psychology, 15,* 166–171.

Klein, S. K., Tuchman, R. F., & Rapin, I. (2000). The influence of premorbid language skills and behavior on language recovery in children with verbal auditory agnosia. *Journal of Child Neurology, 15,* 36–43.

Kraus, N., & McGee, T. (1992). Electrophysiology of the human auditory system. In A. N. Popper & R. R. Fay (Eds.), *The mammalian auditory pathway: Neurophysiology* (pp. 335–403). New York: Springer-Verlag.

Kraus, N., McGee, T., Carrell, T. D., Sharma, A., Koch, D., King, C., et al. (1995). Neurophysiologic bases of speech discrimination. *Ear and Hearing, 16,* 19–37.

Kraus, N., McGee, T., & Comperatore, C. (1990). Middle latency response in sleeping children: Evidence for subcortical contributions to Wave Pa of the human MLR. *ARO Abstracts, 13,* 158.

Kraus, N., McGee, T. J., & Koch, D. B. (1998). Speech sound representation, perception, and plasticity: A neurophysiologic perspective. *Audiology and Neuro-Otology, 3,* 168–182.

Kraus, N., Ozdamar, O., Hier, D., & Stein, L. (1982). Auditory middle latency responses (MLRs) in patients with cortical lesions. *Electroencephalography and Clinical Neurophysiology, 54,* 275–287.

Kulynych, J. J., Vlader, K., Jones, D. W., & Weinberger, D. R. (1994). Gender differences in the normal lateralization of the supratemporal cortex: MRI surface-rendering morphometry of Heschl's gyrus and the planum temporale. *Cerebral Cortex, 4,* 107–118.

Landau, W. M., Goldstein, R., & Kleffner, F. R. (1957). Congenital aphasia: A clinicopathologic study. *Neurology, 7,* 915–921.

Landau, W. M., & Kleffner, F. R. (1957). Syndrome of acquired aphasia with convulsive disorder in children. *Neurology, 7,* 523–530.

Liberman, M. C., & Guinan, J. J. (1998). Feedback control of the auditory periphery: Anti-masking effects of middle ear muscles vs. olivocochlear efferents. *Journal of Communication Disorders, 31,* 471–483.

Maurer, J., Beck, W., Mann, W., & Mintert, R. (1992). Veränderungen otoakustisher Emissionen unto gleichzeitiger

Beschallung des Gegenohres bei Normalpersonen und bei Patientien mit einseitigem Akustikusneurinom. [Changes of amplitude of otoacoustic emissions under contralateral noise in normal hearing persons and in patients with unilateral acoustic neuroma.] *Laryngology-Rhinology-Otology, 71,* 69–73.

McGee, T., & Kraus, N. (1996). Auditory development reflected by middle latency response. *Ear and Hearing, 17,* 419–429.

McPherson, D. L. (1996). *Late potentials of the auditory system.* Clifton Park, NY: Delmar Learning.

Michel, F., Peronnet, F., & Schott, B. (1980). A case of cortical deafness: Clinical and electrophysiological data. *Brain and Language, 10,* 367–377.

Morlet, T., Collet, L., Salle, B., & Morgon, A. (1993). Functional maturation of cochlear active mechanisms and of the medial olivocochlear system in humans. *Acta Otolaryngologica (Stockholm), 113,* 271–277.

Morlet, T., Goforth, L., Hood, L. J., Ferber, C., Duclaux, R., & Berlin, C. I. (1999). Development of human cochlear active mechanism asymmetry: Involvement of the medial olivocochlear system. *Hearing Research, 134,* 153–162.

Naatanen, R., Lehtokoski, A., Lennes, M., Cheour, M., Huotilainen, M., Iivonen, A., et al. (1997). Language-specific phoneme representations revealed by electric and magnetic brain responses. *Nature, 358,* 432–434.

Ozdamar, O., & Kraus, N. (1983). Auditory middle-latency responses in humans. *Audiology, 22,* 34–49.

Ozdamar, O., & Kraus, N., & Curry, F. (1982). Auditory brain stem and middle latency responses in a patient with cortical deafness. *Electroencephalography and Clinical Neurophysiology, 53,* 224–230.

Parving, A., Salomon, G., Elberling, C., Larsen, B., & Lassen, N. A. (1980). Middle components of the auditory evoked response in bilateral temporal lobe lesions. *Scandinavian Audiology, 9,* 161–167.

Penhune, V. B., Zattore, R. J., MacDonald, J. D., & Evans, A. C. (1996). Interhemispheric anatomical differences in human primary auditory cortex: Probabilistic mapping and volume measurement from magnetic resonance scans. *Cerebral Cortex, 6,* 661–672.

Picton, T. W., Hillyard, S. A., Krausz, H. I., & Galambos, R. (1974). Human auditory evoked potentials: I. Evaluation of components. *Electroencephalography and Clinical Neurophysiology, 36,* 179–190.

Ponton, C. W., Don, M., Eggermont, J. J., Waring, M. D., & Masuda, A. (1996). Maturation of human cortical auditory function: Differences between normal-hearing children and children with cochlear implants. *Ear and Hearing, 17,* 430–437.

Rance, G., Beer, D. E., Cone-Wesson, B., Shepherd, R. K., Dowell, R. C., King, A. M., et al. (1999). Clinical findings for a group of infants and young children with auditory neuropathy. *Ear and Hearing, 20,* 238–252.

Ryan, S., Kemp, D. T., & Hinchcliffe, R. (1991). The influence of contralateral acoustic stimulation on click-evoked otoacoustic emissions in humans. *British Journal of Audiology, 25,* 391–397.

Ryan, S., & Piron, J.P. (1994). Functional maturation of the medial olivocochlear system in human neonates. *Acta Otolaryngologica (Stockholm), 114,* 485–489.

Seidenwurm, D., Bird, C. R., Enzmann, D. R., & Marshall, W. H. (1985). Left-right temporal asymmetry in infants and children. *American Journal of Neurology and Radiology, 6,* 777–779.

Starr, A., & Achor, L. J. (1975). Auditory brain stem responses in neurological disease. *Archives of Otolaryngology, 32,* 761–768.

Starr, A., Amlie, R. N., Martin, W. H., & Sanders, S. (1977). Development of auditory function in newborn infants revealed by auditory brainstem potentials. *Pediatrics, 60,* 831–839.

Starr, A., McPherson, D., Patterson, J., Don, M., Luxford, W., Shannon, R., et al. (1991). Absence of both auditory evoked potentials and auditory percepts dependent on timing cues. *Ear and Hearing, 16,* 361–371.

Starr, A., Picton, T. W., Sininger, Y., Hood, L. J., & Berlin, C. I. (1996). Auditory neuropathy. *Brain, 119,* 741–753.

Stein, L., Tremblay, K., Pasternak, J., Banerjee, S., Lindemann, K., & Kraus, N. (1996). Brainstem abnormalities in neonates with normal otoacoustic emissions. *Seminars in Hearing, 17,* 197–213.

Studdert-Kennedy, M., & Shankweiler, D. (1970). Hemispheric specialization for speech perception. *Journal of the Acoustical Society of America, 48,* 579–594.

Syzmanski, M. D., Perry, D. W., Gage, N. M., Rowley, H. A., Walker, J., Berger, M. S., et al. (2001). Magnetic source imaging of late evoked field responses to vowels: Toward an assessment of hemispheric dominance for language. *Journal of Neurosurgery, 94,* 445–453.

Tonnquist-Uhlen, I. (1996). Topography of auditory evoked cortical potentials in children with severe language impairment. *Scandinavian Audiology (Suppl.), 44,* 1–40.

Tremblay, K., Kraus, N., Carrell, T. D., & McGee, T. (1997). Central auditory system plasticity: Generalization to novel stimuli following listening training. *Journal of the Acoustical Society of America, 102,* 3762–3773.

Wada, J. A., Clark, R., & Hamm, A. (1975). Cerebral hemispheric asymmetry in humans: Cortical speech zones in 100 adults and 100 infant brains. *Archives of Neurology, 32,* 239–246.

Wen, H., Berlin, C. I., Hood, L. J., Jackson, D., & Hurley, A. (1993). A program for the quantification and analysis of transient evoked otoacoustic emissions. *ARO Abstracts, 16,* 102.

Williams, E. A., Brookes, G. B., & Prasher, D. K. (1994). Effect of olivocochlear bundle section on otoacoustic emissions in humans: Effects in comparison with control subjects. *Acta Otolaryngologica (Stockholm), 114,* 121–129.

Winkler, I., Lehtokoski, A., Alku, P., Vainio, M., Czigler, I., Csepe, V., et al. (1999). Pre-attentive detection of vowel contrasts utilizes both phonetic and auditory memory representations. *Brain Research Cognition, 7,* 357–369.

Witelson, S. F. (1977). Anatomic asymmetry in the temporal lobes: Its documentation, phylogenesis, and relationship to functional asymmetry. *Annals of the New York Academy of Sciences, 299,* 328–354.

Zeng, F. G., Oba, S., Garde, S., Sininger, Y., & Starr, A. (1999). Temporal processing deficits in auditory neuropathy. *Neuroreport, 10,* 29–35.

7

Fast ForWord™: Its Scientific Basis and Treatment Effects on the Human Efferent Auditory System

Thierry Morlet, Ph.D., Michael Norman,
Beverly Ray, and Charles I. Berlin, Ph.D.
Kresge Hearing Research Laboratory
Louisiana State University Health Sciences Center
New Orleans, LA

ABSTRACT

Chapters 1 and 2, and others in this volume, address theoretical and basic science issues in neural temporal processing across species and systems, and indirectly address plasticity throughout the nervous system. Recently, a powerful and highly effective tool, Fast ForWord™, has been developed and made commercially available. This tool actually trains the temporal and acoustic skill of humans to cope better with rapid transitions of speech and to enhance both comprehension and lexical skills. Fast ForWord™ has been successfully used in some children with central auditory processing disorder (CAPD), specific language impairment (SLI), or attention deficit hyperactivity disorder and their concomitant problems listening in noise. Predicting success and/or candidacy in Fast ForWord™ is important to the field because the program may not be successful for every language-disordered child. Studies of children with SLI show that they present a left ear advantage in efferent auditory suppression, whereas children with normal language skills show a right ear advantage. Furthermore, preliminary studies show that, after successful completion of Fast ForWord™, most SLI children will exhibit a change to a right ear advantage in suppression. Thus, remarkable posttreatment reports and enhanced phonologic awareness and signal-to-noise performance have been reported, which are here linked to physiologic changes recorded by us in efferent suppression of otoacoustic emissions and by others (e.g. Temple et al., 2000) using functional magnetic resonance imaging (fMRI).

SPECIFIC LANGUAGE IMPAIRMENT

There are a significant number of children with language difficulties who have normal sensory, motor, and nonverbal cognitive abilities (Wright et al., 1997). This disorder, known as specific language impairment (SLI), is diagnosed when there is marked impairment in the development of expressive or receptive language that is not associated with mental retardation, autism, hearing impairment, or neurological disorder. The clinical manifestation of SLI can be extremely variable: some children have problems predominantly with production of speech sounds, whereas others make many grammatical errors but appear to understand normally. Children with SLI have difficulties in segmenting, discriminating, and identifying speech sounds (Bishop, 1997). Some authors claim that language impairment arises from failures specific to language or cognitive processing. A matter of controversy is whether such difficulties have their basis in a more fundamental auditory perceptual deficit that affects processing of all sounds, not just speech. Other authors argue that language impairment results from a more elemental problem that makes affected children unable to hear the acoustic distinctions among successive brief sounds in speech.

In children with language disorders, auditory function is usually explored with "classical" audiometry that does not study central functions either afferent or efferent especially with respect to hearing in noise. There are two distinct efferent auditory pathways between the brain and the cochlea (Rasmussen, 1946; Warr & Guinan, 1979), implying that the acoustic signal stimulating the cochlea can be modified before it reaches the brain. The first population of efferent neurons, thin and unmyelinated, arises from the lateral superior olivary complex and synapses with cochlear afferent neuron dendrites, beneath inner hair cells (IHCs) that are the primary, sensory receptors of the auditory system. The second population of neurons, known as the medial olivocochlear system (MOCS), is composed of large myelinated neurons originating from the medial nuclei of the superior olivary complex. These neurons project both ipsilaterally and contralaterally to innervate outer hair cells (OHCs), which are presumably the source of cochlear active mechanisms (Brownell, Bader, Bertrand, & de Ribeaupierre, 1985). This system seems to be involved in the detection of signals in noise (Micheyl & Collet, 1995; Micheyl, Morlet, Girand, Collet, & Morgon, 1995; Winslow & Sachs, 1987), such as speech sounds (Giraud et al., 1997), by modulating the cochlear active mechanisms (CAMs). Otoacoustic emissions (OAEs) are thought to be the by-products of CAM, that is, the activity of OHCs (Brownell et al., 1985; Kemp, 1978). Evidence of CAM modulation by the MOCS comes mainly from numerous studies on OAEs. As a matter of fact, in the 1990s, experiments indicated the possibility of studying the MOCS' activity noninvasively in adults by coupling a contralateral acoustic stimulation to OAE recording (Berlin et al., 1993; Collet et al., 1990; Ryan, Kemp, & Hinchcliffe, 1991; Veuillet, Collet, & Duclaux, 1991).

This study's hypothesis regarding children with SLI was that despite normal "classical" audiological findings, they might have an impaired efferent auditory function that would lead to difficulties in processing speech, mainly under noisy conditions. The first study addressed this question by studying MOCS function and auditory brain stem responses in a group of 16 SLI children aged from 5 to 10 years old matched to a group of 15 children with normal language functioning.

The language disordered participants were identified by a speech-language pathologist who completed a speech and language assessment battery, including the Clinical Evaluation of Language Fundamentals, third edition (CELF-3). CELF-3 provides three norm-referenced composite scores. The CELF-3 Total Language score quantifies the overall language performance. The Receptive Language score reflects the ability to process and understand verbal communication. The Expressive Language score reflects the ability to express verbally. Children in the control group were known to have normal hearing, intelligence, and speech and language development. They were selected from families of colleagues and friends and matched with the SLI children for age. None of those children had a history of significant middle-ear disease or any known medical problems. Written parental consent was obtained for each child involved in the experiment.

To investigate the MOCS function, transient evoked otoacoustic emissions (TEOAEs) were recorded using ILO88 from Otodynamics. Efferent suppression of TEOAEs was studied in both ears using a forward masking procedure (Berlin, Hood, Hurley, Wen, & Kemp, 1995), allowing ipsilateral, contralateral, and binaural noise stimulation. Linear clicks at a 63 ± 3 dB sound pressure level (SPL) intensity level were presented to elicit TEOAEs. A 400-msec white noise (at 65 dB SPL) was used to stimulate the MOCS. The interval between the offset of the noise and the onset of the click was set at 10 msec. Two recordings of TEOAEs without noise were interleaved with one TEOAE recording for each noise condition, that is, ipsilateral, contralateral, and binaural. The order of noise presentation was randomly selected. The analysis time was 20 msec with the initial 2.5 msec software-zeroed to eliminate the stimulus artifact. The ear-canal signal was band-pass filtered from 0.5 to 6 kHz. One hundred responses were averaged for each recording two times.

The auditory brain stem responses (ABRs) were recorded in both ears with monaural and binaural stimulation using the CHARTR system from ICS Medical Corp. The positive electrode was located at Cz and the negative electrodes on each ear lobe. The ground electrode was placed on the forehead. Condensation clicks (100-μsec duration) were presented at a rate of 21.1/sec through insert earphones. The sweep time was 15 msec, including a delay prestimulus of 3 msec. In this study, 2,000 sweeps were averaged, and the recording was repeated twice for each condition. The gain was set at 100K, with low-frequency filtering at 50 Hz and high-frequency filtering at 3 kHz. Clicks were presented at 75 dB and 50 dB hearing level re: a normal jury (nHL). Children were allowed to watch a silent movie on a monitor inside the booth to keep them as still as possible. Right and left ears were tested in random order for both TEOAE and ABR recordings.

Suppression was determined by subtracting the without-contralateral stimulation (CS) condition from the with-CS condition using the Kresge EchoMaster emission analysis program version 3.11 (Wen, Berlin, Hood, & Jackson, 1993) (see a detailed explanation in Hood, chapter 6 of this volume). The latencies of the brain stem auditory evoked potentials were obtained for waves I, III, and V. Peak-to-following-trough amplitudes were measured for waves I, III, and V. Repeated analysis of variance (ANOVA) measures were used to compare root-mean-square (RMS) suppression and TEOAE amplitudes between right ears (RE) and left ears (LE). One-way ANOVA was used to compare both groups. When the ANOVA reached significance, post hoc analyses were completed with the Tukey test.

SLI children presented normal ABRs in terms of wave latencies and amplitudes (see Tables 7-1 to 7-3). In those children as well as in controls, no specific asymmetry of ABR was noticed. Although several authors found ABR abnormalities in children with learning problems, speech and language disorders, and auditory processing deficit, several did not (Marosi, Harmony, & Becker, 1990) or did with amplitudes but not latencies (Mason & Mellor, 1984).

Table 7-1 Absolute Latency (msec) of the ABRs (mean ± s.e.)

	I		III		V	
	LE	RE	LE	RE	LE	RE
SLI	1.30	1.36	3.52	3.54	5.41	5.40
	(0.02)	(0.03)	(0.04)	(0.04)	(0.03)	(0.04)
Control	1.20	1.29	3.42	3.40	5.37	5.40
	(0.04)	(0.04)	(0.13)	(0.12)	(0.06)	(0.09)

Table 7-2 Interwave Latency (msec) of the ABR (mean ± s.e.)

	I–III		III–V		I–V	
	LE	RE	LE	RE	LE	RE
SLI	2.23	2.18	1.88	1.87	4.11	4.05
	(0.04)	(0.04)	(0.04)	(0.03)	(0.05)	(0.05)
Control	2.20	2.13	1.95	1.94	4.17	4.10
	(0.11)	(0.12)	(0.07)	(0.06)	(0.04)	(0.08)

Table 7-3 Amplitude (µV) of the ABR (mean ± s.e.)

	I		III		V	
	LE	RE	LE	RE	LE	RE
SLI	0.21	0.22	0.17	0.19	0.58	0.66
	(0.03)	(0.04)	(0.02)	(0.02)	(0.06)	(0.06)
Control	0.34	0.24	0.14	0.14	0.47	0.50
	(0.06)	(0.04)	(0.05)	(0.04)	(0.05)	(0.05)

TEOAEs were present in all SLI and control children. In both groups, TEOAEs were considered normal in terms of amplitude and spectral contents. In both groups, TEOAE amplitude was found to be significantly higher in the RE than in the LE. TEOAE overall amplitude obtained without suppressor, however, was found to be significantly lower in SLI children than normals in both ears (Figure 7-1).

The MOCS function appeared to be present in all the children with SLI, and a substantial variability in the amount of TEOAE suppression was observed. The variability of suppression, however, seems to be a common feature among various populations of neonates, children, and adults (Hamburger, Ari-Even Roth, Muchnik, Kuint, & Hildesheimer, 1998; Hood, Berlin, Hurley, Cecola, & Bell, 1996; Morlet et al., 1999; Veuillet et al., 1991). These children behaved like normal in that they showed a greater suppression effect for binaurally presented stimuli than for ipsilaterally or contralaterally presented stimuli (Berlin et al., 1995).

Recordings of TEOAE suppression, however, have indicated higher efferent suppression in the left than the right ear in the SLI group (Figure 7-2). The MOCS function is known to be more efficient in the RE than the LE among the normal hearing population (Khalfa & Collet, 1996; Khalfa, Morlet, Micheyl, Morgon, & Collet, 1997). This fact was verified among the control children for the bilateral condition, even if the difference did not reach significance due to the low number of subjects.

This study shows that children with SLI present some subtle auditory differences with normal subjects. The main finding is that children with SLI show higher efferent suppression of TEOAEs in the LE than in the RE. The MOCS appears to be more efficient in RE than in LE in normal adults (Khalfa & Collet, 1996) and neonates

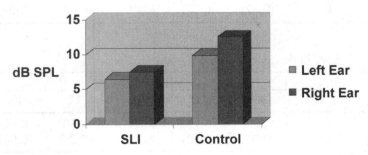

Figure 7-1. TEOAE overall amplitude in children with SLI and in normal children.

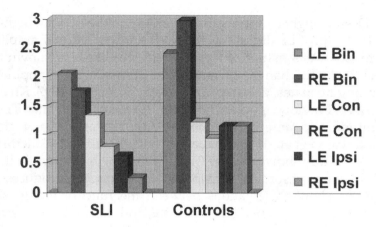

Figure 7-2. Suppression of TEOAEs following binaural, contralateral, and ipsilateral stimulations in SLI and control children.

(Morlet et al., 1999). This asymmetrical feature is suggested (McFadden, 1993) to be closely related to the greater hearing sensitivity in the RE than in the LE (Glorig, 1958; Pirilä, 1991). The RE advantage is supposed to be in relation with the language function, lateralized to the left hemisphere (Chi, Dooling, & Gilles, 1977). As a matter of fact, signals from each ear reach both temporal lobes, but crossed pathways have more fibers and produce more cortical activity than uncrossed ones. Thus, the right ear advantage (REA) is usually interpreted as a result of the dominance of the left hemisphere for processing speech and language and of the inhibition of ipsilateral auditory pathways. Several anatomical and functional asymmetries from the cochlea to the cortex are evidence in support of the REA. At the cochlear level, there are significant differences in transient OAE (TEOAE) amplitude between both ears (Kei, McPherson, Smyth, Latham, & Tallal, 1997; Khalfa et al., 1997). In adults, infants, and both full-term and preterm neonates, spontaneous OAEs are found more often in the RE than in the LE (Burns, Hoberg, Arehart, & Campbell, 1992; Kok, van Zanten, & Brocaar, 1993; Morlet et al., 1995). Asymmetries are observed along the afferent pathways as well as for the efferent fibers. Indeed, the MOCS appears to be more efficient in the RE than in the LE (Khalfa & Collet, 1996).

The MOCS function, however, does not seem to be strictly the opposite between SLI and control groups. The amount of suppression measured in both groups suggests that the higher suppression in the LE than in the RE in SLI children is rather due to a lower functioning of the MOCS in the RE.

Despite higher suppression of TEOAE in the LE than in the RE, children with SLI did show the well-known TEOAE amplitude asymmetry. As a matter of fact, TEOAE amplitude is known to be higher in the RE than the LE among the normal hearing population, including neonates, children, and adults (Kei et al., 1997; Khalfa et al., 1997). Previous studies, however, have reported that TEOAE amplitude and amount of efferent suppression are not closely related (Hood et al., 1996; Khalfa, Micheyl, Veuillet, & Collet, 1998).

This study shows that the MOCS function in children with specific language disorders is impaired. This result introduces new questions about the relations between the functional role of the MOCS, the greater sensitivity of the RE, and the auditory lateralization needed to develop and process speech. It has been found that SLI is related to abnormal asymmetries of perisylvian regions of the temporal lobe with an absence of a greater left than right perisylvian region (Plante, Swisher, Vance, & Rapcsak, 1991). Other asymmetrical differences have been found in the prefrontal, inferior, posterior, and superior temporal cortex (Jernigan, Hesselilnk, Sowell, & Tallal, 1991). SLI children are thought to be having problems in processing rapid sequences of brief sounds (Cacace & McFarland, 1998; Lubert, 1981). They would thus be unable to detect rapid transitions that occur between phonemes. They need longer neural processing time between brief, successive acoustic signals than normally developing children so as to process them. This slower processing rate causes the child problems when attempting to distinguish speech sounds within the 10-msec window.

TREATING AND MANAGING CHILDREN WITH SLI OR CENTRAL AUDITORY DISORDERS

Fast ForWord™ is a very powerful neuroscience-based treatment for some forms of SPI, CAPD, or phonological disorders, especially those accompanied by histories of auditory deprivation. These children also are described as having problems hearing in noise. In part because of its expense and in part because of schools opting for less expensive "similar" programs, being able to predict when and if the Fast ForWord™ system will outperform others is very useful. Because, according to some professionals, Fast ForWord™ does not always work as predicted or hoped for, having a physiologic predictor or an index of potential success is quite important to conserve resources and justify the procedure to third-party payors. This chapter explains the theory of Fast ForWord™, how and why it works on the patients it does help, and what physiologic changes are demonstrated in efferent function (this research on almost 50 children) and cortical function via fMRI (Temple et al.'s recent research on almost 30 other schoolchildren in the *Proceedings of the National Academy of Science*). A number of tutorials are available on the enclosed CD-ROM and from www.scilearn.com.

SOME OF THE TEMPORAL BUILDING BLOCKS OF SPEECH PERCEPTION

The acoustic building blocks of speech can be examined in the three dimensions of frequency, intensity, and time. A simple sine wave then can be displayed in three different manners (see Figures 7-3, 7-4 and 7-5 and accompanying CD-ROM).

The ability of the normal auditory system to detect and process these signals has been well studied. For example, the frequency range of human hearing is from about 20 Hz to about 18 kHz by air conduction but about 60 kHz via bone conduction, although tonal discrimination and sensation drop off below 20 Hz and above 18 kHz. The human ear can detect changes of less than 1 dB when the

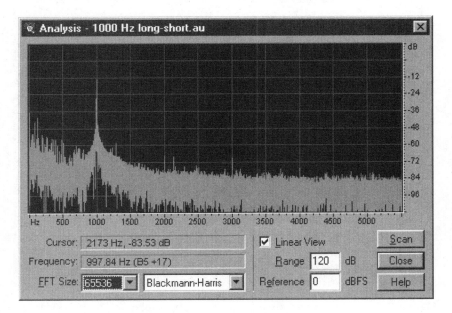

Figure 7-3. Frequency-by-time display of a 1000-Hz tone.

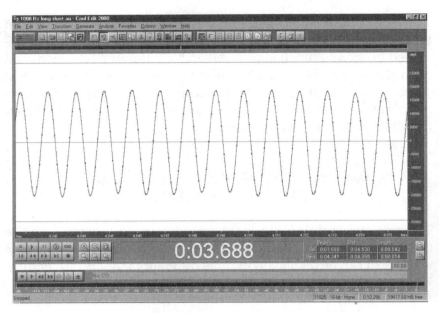

Figure 7-4. Amplitude-by-time display of a 1000-Hz tone.

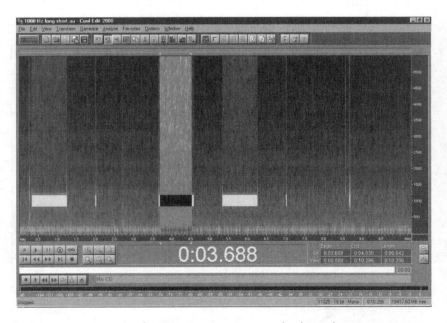

Figure 7-5. A time-by-frequency spectrogram display of a 1000-Hz tone repeated seven times and lengthened and shortened for clarification.

stimulus is more than 70 dB but needs more intensity to detect fainter sounds. What is particularly interesting to the topic today is how well the human ear must function to detect small changes in acoustic intervals and temporal pattern directions and how well the brain must function to categorize, store, and recall these brief temporal patterns. Some, but not all, of our language comprehension, storage, retrieval, and use hinges on the temporal processes of speech perception. In the enclosed disk are examples of time-by-frequency patterns of speech that elicit certain perceptions in most normal listeners. The disk also shows in part how Fast ForWord™ can train the auditory system to improve its performance and enhance its ability to detect small changes under noisy conditions.

Here is an example of two synthetic utterances a /ba/ and a /pa/ (Figures 7-6 and 7-7). They differ only at the beginning, where the /pa/ shows a long noise burst that is absent in the /ba/.

The accompanying disk gives examples of speech analysis and shows how failure to perceive key elements, especially of the second formant (see Sussman, chapter 2 of this volume) and the brain's inability to detect gaps and sequences in the speech stream, can lead to serious language and speech problems. A series of neural plasticity–based games is offered in Fast ForWord™, samples of which are available from www.scilearn.com. This demonstration disk also

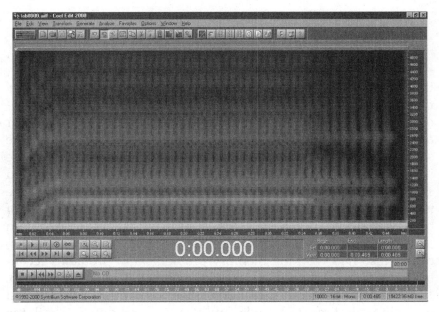

Figure 7-6. A synthetic utterance leading to a perception of /ba/.

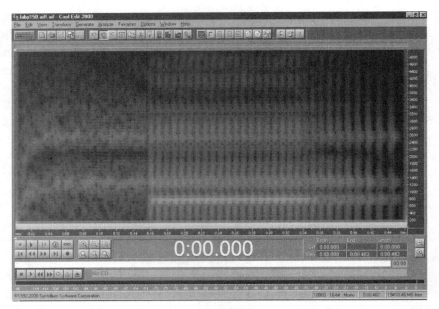

Figure 7-7. A synthetic utterance inducing the perception of /pa/ in a normal listener.

explains which building blocks of speech and language are being trained and how and why the training builds neural connections.

A BRIEF SYNOPSIS OF THE HISTORY OF FAST FORWORD™ AND TEMPORAL PROCESSING DISORDERS

In the early 1960s, a classical set of papers by Robert Efron showed that aphasics with (usually) left temporal lobe disorders had serious difficulties managing temporal sequences in either visual or auditory modalities. Gap detection and sequence detection were soon thereafter found to be abnormal in children with language impairment (e.g., Lowe & Campbell, 1965). In closely connected studies, Tallal and Piercy (1973, 1974, 1975) showed that language impaired children were poorer at managing temporal sequences of both verbal and nonverbal stimuli as well as synthetic speech stimuli. This group at Kresge showed children with language disorders also had working memory problems and problems recalling two dichotic stimuli in sequence (Tobey, Cullen, & Rampp, 1979; Tobey, Fleischer-Gallagher, Cullen, & Rampp, 1982). Based on their earliest research, Tallal and Piercy concluded that both the duration of the consonant and the speed of the transition were critical to successful performance of children with language impairment. Tallal, Miller, and Fitch (1993) summarized these studies with the notion that children with language impairment have poor auditory processing skills and that remediation of the auditory processing difficulty should lead to improvement in language comprehension and expression.

Fast ForWord™ was launched when Merzenich et al. (1996) and Tallal et al. (1996) showed that acoustically modified speech stimuli can assist school-age children with presumably *auditorily based* language learning disorders (reviewed in Merzenich, Tallal, Peterson, Miller, & Jenkins, 1999). Stressed here is "auditorily based" because some children with language or reading disorders that are *not* auditorily based do not benefit from Fast ForWord™. This point is important because in a recent monograph, Friel-Patti, Loeb, and Gillam (2001) present what they believed to be a balanced assessment of Fast ForWord™ efficacy, but did not choose the children based on any temporal processing tasks. Very complete verbal descriptions of the exercises, however, can be found on pages 197–198 of their monograph. The games and their rationales can also be seen in demonstration disks at www.scilearn.com.

Thus, Fast ForWord™ assumes that rapid auditory processing is at risk in these children and that a systematic neuroscience-based training program can help reorganize their nervous systems in much the same way Merzenich and colleagues were able to retrain monkey somatosensory and motor systems after injury (Merzenich et al., 1984; Wright et al., 1997). The developers of Fast ForWord™ created the following games and tasks:

- Circus Sequence (CS): The subject has to discriminate between a sequence of two brief successive acoustic sweeps that are separated by a specified interstimulus interval.
- Old McDonald's Flying Farm (OMDFF): The subject has to distinguish sound changes at the level of individual phonemes.
- Phoneme Identification (PI): The subject has to identify specific phonemes.
- Phonic Match (PM): This task reinforces memory and reasoning skills within simple word structures that differ by a single phoneme.
- Phonic Words (PW): The subject has to distinguish between words that differed only by either an initial or final consonant.

- Language Comprehension Builder (LCB): This task introduces increasingly complex sentences to develop higher-level language skills, including phonology, morphology, syntax, and grammar.
- Block Commander (BC): The subject is taught listening comprehension and syntax and is trained in short-term memory through the use of complex sentence structures.

The children studied clearly have auditory anomalies that reveal themselves via abnormalities in the brain stem–mediated medial olivocochlear reflex.

This ongoing study is investigating if MOCS function is changing over time in relation with an improvement of language skills in SLI children undergoing 8 weeks of speech therapy. Two groups of children (SLI and normal) are studied. Both groups are going through Fast ForWord™ concurrently. The clinical evaluation of the CELF-3 test is administered to both groups before and after the Fast ForWord™ training, and recordings of the MOCS function are made as well. Preliminary results show that improvement of language skills (Figure 7-8) is concomitant with an increase of MOCS function. Both functions increased after training. The MOCS function was found to augment more in the right ear than the left ear. After training, MOCS function tended to normalize with a right ear advantage.

OTHER PHYSIOLOGICAL EVIDENCE

In the course of evaluating children for CAPD, it has been our practice to rule out auditory neuropathy (see Berlin et al., 2002)

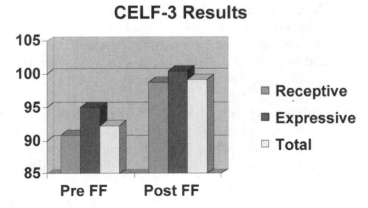

Figure 7-8. CELF-3 results before and after Fast ForWord™ in SLI children, showing an improvement of language skills.

and then study the children with a special version of middle latency responses (MLR). The rationale for this study came from Hood, Martin, and Berlin (1990), who showed that right-handed and left handed people had different MLR responses at Pb, where the left-handed subjects responded at 55 msecs, whereas the right-handed subjects responded at 50 msecs. This finding is considered a physiological marker of interhemispheric transfer, which would enable researchers to gain insight into how the brains of these children were organized vis-á-vis their handedness. The main difference between this technique and standard technique is that the stimulation rate has to be 3 per second or slower, in contrast to the more common 7 per second or faster. It was found that the majority of the children studied showed no Pb or a Pb in the "wrong place," but that after successful treatment with Fast ForWord™ their MLRs normalized. A pre- and post-Fast ForWord™ sample is seen in Figure 7-9.

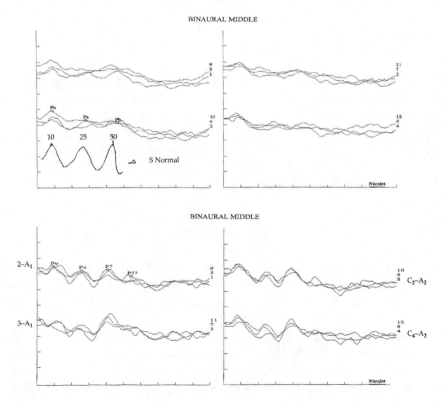

Figure 7-9. An example of MLRs in a child with CAPD recorded before and after completion of Fast ForWord™.

There is insufficient data on untreated normals or different controls to be sure that this finding is not simply maturation or the effects of learning in general rather than Fast ForWord™ in particular, but current research is studying the use of MLR as both a pre- and post-Fast ForWord™ test.

Poldrack and colleagues (2001) and Temple and colleagues (2001) have recently shown dramatic changes in fMRI after Fast ForWord™. They have shown that dyslexic subjects who listen to synthetic speech utterances with slow versus fast consonant-like onsets differ markedly from normals. The normal brain responds more vigorously to the fast-onset stimuli that emulate speech in the left frontal areas and right cerebellar areas. The dyslexic brain shows little if any lateralization to any of these stimuli but responds more vigorously in the midline to the slow-onset stimuli than the fast-onset stimuli. This finding suggests that temporal onset is not clearly marked in dyslexic brains and that failure to perceive consonantal onsets or intervals may be one of the underlying bases of auditory-based dyslexia or language problems.

CONCLUSIONS

Physiologic changes after Fast ForWord™ reflect plasticity in the human nervous system. Whether these changes occur after other regimens was not investigated here, but that learning leads to changes in the brain is agreed upon by any and all investigators. These are exciting times in which neuroscience findings are being applied to human language and communication problems in ways that have never before been possible.

REFERENCES

Berlin, C. I., Hood, L. J., Hurley, A. E., Wen, H., & Kemp, D. T. (1995). Binaural noise suppresses linear click-evoked otoacoustic emissions more than ipsilateral or contralateral noise. *Hearing Research, 87,* 96–103.

Berlin, C. I., Hood, L. J., Jeanfreau, J., Morlet, T., Brashears, S., & Keats, B. (2002). The physiological bases of audiological management. In C. I. Berlin, L. J. Hood, & A. Ricci (Eds.), *Hair cell micromechanics and otoacoustic emissons* (pp. 139–154). Clifton Park, NY: Delmar.

Berlin, C. I., Hood, L. J., Wen, H., Szabo, P., Cecola, R. P., Rigby, P., et al. (1993). Contralateral suppression of non-linear click-evoked otoacoustic emissions. *Hearing Research, 71,* 1–11.

Bishop, D. V. (1997). Language impairment: Listening out for subtle deficits. *Nature, 387,* 129–130.

Brownell, W. E., Bader, C. R., Bertrand, D., & de Ribeaupierre, Y. (1985). Evoked mechanical responses of isolated cochlear hair cells. *Science, 227,* 194–196.

Burns, E. M., Hoberg, R., Arehart, K., & Campbell, S. L. (1992). Prevalence of spontaneous otoacoustic emissions in neonates. *Journal of the Acoustical Society of America, 91,* 1571–1575.

Cacace, A. T., & McFarland D. J. (1998). Central auditory processing disorder in school-aged children: A critical review. *Journal of Speech, Languages, and Hearing Research, 41,* 355–373.

Chi, J. G., Dooling, E. C., & Gilles, F. H. (1977). Left-right asymmetries of the temporal speech areas of the human fetus. *Archives of Neurology, 34,* 346–348.

Collet, L., Kemp, D. T., Veuillet, E., Duclaux, R., Moulin, A., & Morgon, A. (1990). Effect of contralateral auditory stimuli on active cochlear micro-mechanical properties in human subjects. *Hearing Research, 43,* 251–262.

Friel-Patti, S., Loeb, D. F., & Gillam, R. B. (2001). Looking ahead: An introduction to five exploratory studies of Fast ForWard. *American Journal of Speech-Language Pathology, 10*(3), 195–202.

Giraud, A. L., Garnier, S., Micheyl, C., Lina, G., Chays, A., & Chery-Croze, S. (1997). Auditory efferents involved in speech-in-noise intelligibility. *Neuroreport, 8,* 1779–1783.

Glorig, A. (1958). A report of two normal hearing studies. *Annals of Otology, Rhinology, and Laryngology, 67,* 93–111.

Hamburger, A., Ari-Even Roth, D., Muchnik, C., Kuint, J., & Hildesheimer, M. (1998). Contralateral acoustic effect of transient evoked otoacoustic emissions in neonates. *International Tinnitus Journal, 4,* 53–57.

Hood, L. J., Berlin, C. I., Hurley, A., Cecola, R. P., & Bell, B. (1996). Contralateral suppression of transient-evoked otoacoustic emissions in humans: Intensity effects. *Hearing Research, 101,* 113–118.

Hood, L. J., Martin, D. A., & Berlin, C. I. (1990). Auditory evoked potentials differ at 50 milliseconds in right- and left-handed listeners. *Hearing Research, 45,* 115–122.

Jernigan, T. L., Hesselilnk, J. R., Sowell, E., & Tallal, P. A. (1991). Cerebral structure on magnetic resonance imaging in language- and learning-impaired children. *Archives of Neurology, 48,* 539–545.

Kei, J., McPherson, B., Smyth, V., Latham, S., & Loscher, J. (1997). Transient evoked otoacoustic emissions in infants: Effects of gender, ear asymmetry and activity status. *Audiology, 36,* 61–71.

Kemp, D. T. (1978). Stimulated acoustic emissions from within the human auditory system. *Journal Acoustical Society America, 64,* 1386–1391.

Khalfa, S., & Collet, L. (1996). Functional asymmetry of medial olivocochlear system in humans: Towards a peripheral auditory lateralization. *Neuroreport, 7,* 993–996.

Khalfa, S., Micheyl, C., Veuillet, E., & Collet, L. (1998). Peripheral auditory lateralization assessment using TEOAEs. *Hearing Research, 121,* 29–34.

Khalfa, S., Morlet, T., Micheyl, C., Morgon, A., & Collet, L. (1997). Evidence for peripheral hearing asymmetry in humans: Clinical implications. *Acta Otolaryngologica (Stockholm), 17,* 192–196.

Kok, M. R., van Zanten, G. A., & Brocaar, M. P. (1993). Aspects of spontaneous otoacoustic emissions in healthy newborns. *Hearing Research, 69,* 115–123.

Lowe, A. D., & Campbell, R. A. (1965). Temporal discrimination in aphasoid and normal children. *Journal Speech Hearing Research, 8,* 313–314.

Lubert, N. (1981). Auditory perceptual impairments in children with specific language disorders: A review of the literature. *Journal of Speech and Hearing Disorders, 46,* 3–9.

Marosi, E., Harmony, T., & Becker, E. (1990). Brainstem evoked potentials in learning disabled children. *International Journal of Neuroscience, 50,* 233–242.

Mason, S. M., & Mellor, D. H. (1984) Brain-stem, middle latency and late cortical evoked potentials in children with speech and language disorders. *Electroencephalography and Clinical Neurophysiology, 59,* 297–309.

McFadden, D. (1993). A speculation about the parallel ear asymmetries and sex differences in hearing sensitivity and otoacoustic emissions. *Hearing Research, 68,* 143–151.

Merzenich, M. M., Jenkins, W., Johnston, P., Schreiner, C., Miller, S. L., & Tallal, P. (1996). Temporal processing deficits of language-learning impaired children ameliorated by training. *Science, 271,* 77–81.

Merzenich, M. M., Nelson, R. J., Stryker, M. P., Cynader, M. S., Schoppmann, A., & Zook, J. M. (1984). Somatosensory cortical map changes following digit amputation in adult monkeys. *Journal of Comparative Neurology, 224*(4), 591–605.

Merzenich, M. M., Tallal P., Peterson B., Miller S., & Jenkins W. M. (1999). Some neurological principles relevant to the origins of— and the cortical plasticity-based remediation of—developmental language impairments. In J. Grafman & Y. Christen (Eds.), *Neuronal plasticity: Building a bridge from the laboratory to the clinic.* New York: Springer-Verlag.

Micheyl, C., & Collet, L. (1995). Involvement of medial olivo-cochlear system in the detection of tones in noise. *Journal of the Acoustical Society of America, 99,* 1604–1610.

Micheyl, C., Morlet, T., Giraud, A. L., Collet, L., & Morgon, A. (1995). Contralateral suppression of evoked otoacoustic emissions and detection of a multitone complex in noise. *Acta Otolaryngologica (Stockholm), 115,* 178–182.

Morlet, T., Goforth, L., Hood, L. J., Ferber, C., Duclaux, R., & Berlin, C. I. (1999). Development of human cochlear active mechanisms asymmetry: Involvement of the medial olivocochlear system? *Hearing Research, 134,* 153–162.

Morlet, T., Lapillonne, A., Ferber, C., Duclaux, R., Sann, L., Putet, G. et al. (1995). Spontaneous otoacoustic emissions in preterm neonates: Prevalence and gender effect. *Hearing Research, 90,* 44–54.

Pirilä, T. (1991). Interaural hearing threshold asymmetry: Epidemiological and experimental studies. *Acta Universitatis Ouluensis, Series D. medica,* 220.

Plante, E., Swisher, L., Vance, R., & Rapcsak, S. (1991). MRI findings in boys with specific language impairment. *Brain and Language, 41,* 52–66.

Poldrack, R. A., Temple, E., Protopapas, A., Nagarajan, S., Tallal, P., Merzenich, M., et al. (2001). Relations between the neural bases of dynamic auditory processing and phonological processing: Evidence from fMRI. *Journal of Cognitive Neuroscience, 13*(5), 687–697.

Rasmussen, G. L. (1946). The olivary peduncle and other fiber projections of the superior olivary complex. *Journal of Comparative Neurology, 84,* 141–218.

Ryan, S., Kemp, D. T., & Hinchcliffe, R. (1991). The influence of contralateral auditory stimulation on otoacoustic emission responses in humans. *British Journal of Audiology, 25,* 391–397.

Tallal, P., Miller, S. L., Bedi, G., Byma, G., Wang, X., Nagarajan, S. S., et al. (1996). Language comprehension in language-learning impaired children improved with acoustically modified speech. *Science, 271,* 81–84.

Tallal, P., Miller, S., & Fitch, R. H. (1993). Neurobiological basis of speech: A case for the preeminence of temporal processing. *Annals of the New York Academy of Science, 14*(682), 27–47.

Tallal, P., & Piercy, M. (1973). Defects of non-verbal auditory perception in children with developmental aphasia. *Nature, 16*(241), 468–469.

Tallal, P., & Piercy, M. (1974). Developmental aphasia: Rate of auditory processing and selective impairment of consonant perception. *Neuropsychologia, 12,* 83–93.

Tallal, P., & Piercy, M. (1975). Developmental aphasia: The perception of brief vowels and extended stop consonants. *Neuropsychologia, 13,* 69–74.

Temple, E., Poldrack, R. A., Protopapas, A., Nagarajan, S., Slaz, T., Merzenich, M. M., et al. (2000). Disruption of the neural response to rapid acoustic stimuli in dyslexia: Evidence from functional MRI. *Proceedings of the National Academy of Science, 97,* 13907–13912.

Temple, E., Poldrack, R. A., Salidis, J., Deutsch, G. K., Tallal, P., Merzenich, M. M., et al. (2001). Disrupted neural responses to phonological and orthographic processing in dyslexic children: An fMRI study. *Neuroreport, 12,* 299–307.

Tobey, E. A., Cullen, J. K., Jr., & Rampp, D. L. (1979). Effects of stimulus-onset asynchrony on the dichotic performance of children with auditory-processing disorders. *Journal of Speech and Hearing Research, 22,* 197–211.

Tobey, E. A., Fleischer-Gallagher, A., Cullen, J. K., Jr., & Rampp, D. L. (1982). Recall performance of children failing memory portions of a speech-language-memory screening battery. *Journal of Communication Disorders, 15,* 259–273.

Veuillet, E., Collet, L., & Duclaux, R. (1991). Effect of contralateral acoustic stimulation on active cochlear micromechanical properties in human subjects: Dependence on stimulus variables. *Journal of Neurophysiology, 65,* 724–735.

Warr, W. B., & Guinan, J. J., Jr. (1979). Efferent innervation of the organ of Corti: Two separate systems. *Brain Research, 173,* 152–155.

Wen, H., Berlin, C. I., Hood, L. J., & Jackson, D. (1993). A program for the quantification and analysis of transient evoked otoacoustic emissions. *Abstracts of the Association for Research in Otolaryngology,* 102.

Winslow, R. L., & Sachs, M. B. (1987). Effect of electrical stimulation of the crossed olivocochlear bundle on auditory nerve response to tones in noise. *Journal Neurophysiology, 57,* 1002–1021.

Wright, B. A., Lombardino, L. J., King, W. M., Puranik, C. S., Leonard, C. M., & Merzenich, M. M. (1997). Deficits in auditory temporal and spectral resolution in language-impaired children. *Nature, 8,* 176–178.

Index

License Agreement for Delmar Learning, a division of Thomson Learning, Inc.

Educational Software/Data

You the customer, and Delmar Learning, a division of Thomson Learning, Inc. incur certain benefits, rights, and obligations to each other when you open this package and use the software/data it contains. BE SURE YOU READ THE LICENSE AGREEMENT CAREFULLY, SINCE BY USING THE SOFTWARE/DATA YOU INDICATE YOU HAVE READ, UNDERSTOOD, AND ACCEPTED THE TERMS OF THIS AGREEMENT.

Your rights:

1. You enjoy a non-exclusive license to use the software/data on a single microcomputer in consideration for payment of the required license fee, (which may be included in the purchase price of an accompanying print component), or receipt of this software/data, and your acceptance of the terms and conditions of this agreement.

2. You acknowledge that you do not own the aforesaid software/data. You also acknowledge that the software/data is furnished "as is," and contains copyrighted and/or proprietary and confidential information of Delmar Learning, a division of Thomson Learning, Inc. or its licensors.

There are limitations on your rights:

1. You may not copy or print the software/data for any reason whatsoever, except to install it on a hard drive on a single microcomputer and to make one archival copy, unless copying or printing is expressly permitted in writing or statements recorded on the diskette(s).

2. You may not revise, translate, convert, disassemble or otherwise reverse engineer the software/data except that you may add to or rearrange any data recorded on the media as part of the normal use of the software/data.

3. You may not sell, license, lease, rent, loan or otherwise distribute or network the software/data except that you may give the software/data to a student or and instructor for use at school or, temporarily at home.

Should you fail to abide by the Copyright Law of the United States as it applies to this software/data your license to use it will become invalid. You agree to erase or otherwise destroy the software/data immediately after receiving note of termination of this agreement for violation of its provisions from Delmar Learning.

Delmar Learning, a division of Thomson Learning, Inc gives you a LIMITED WARRANTY covering the enclosed software/data. The LIMITED WARRANTY follows this License.

This license is the entire agreement between you and Delmar Learning, a division of Thomson Learning, Inc. interpreted and enforced under New York law.

LIMITED WARRANTY

Delmar Learning, a division of Thomson Learning, Inc. warrants to the original licensee/purchaser of this copy of microcomputer software/data and the media on which it is recorded that the media will be free from defects in material and workmanship for ninety (90) days from the date of original purchase. All implied warranties are limited in duration to this ninety (90) day period. THEREAFTER, ANY IMPLIED WARRANTIES, INCLUDING IMPLIED WARRANTIES OF MERCHANTABILITY AND FITNESS FOR A PARTICULAR PURPOSE, ARE EXCLUDED. THIS WARRANTY IS IN LIEU OF ALL OTHER WARRANTIES, WHETHER ORAL OR WRITTEN, EXPRESS OR IMPLIED.

If you believe the media is defective please return it during the ninety day period to the address shown below. Defective media will be replaced without charge provided that it has not been subjected to misuse or damage.

This warranty does not extend to the software or information recorded on the media. The software and information are provided "AS IS." Any statements made about the utility of the software or information are not to be considered as express or implied warranties.

Limitation of liability: Our liability to you for any losses shall be limited to direct damages, and shall not exceed the amount you paid for the software. In no event will we be liable to you for any indirect, special, incidental, or consequential damages (including loss of profits) even if we have been advised of the possibility of such damages.

Some states do not allow the exclusion or limitation of incidental or consequential damages, or limitations on the duration of implied warranties, so the above limitation or exclusion may not apply to you. This warranty gives you specific legal rights, and you may also have other rights which vary from state to state. Address all correspondence to: Delmar Learning, a division of Thomson Learning, Inc., 5 Maxwell Drive, P.O. Box 8007, Clifton Park, NY 12065-8007. Attention: Technology Department

THE BRAIN AND SENSORY PLASTICITY: LANGUAGE ACQUISITION AND HEARING

SYSTEM REQUIREMENTS

Windows® 98 or later

32 MB RAM

800 x 600 display with 16-bit or 64000 colors

12x CD-ROM Drive

Windows-compatible sound card

To view the Microsoft® PowerPoint® and Word documents included on this CD-ROM, you will need the Microsoft® PowerPoint® and Microsoft® Word programs. If you do not have these programs installed on your system, you may use the PowerPoint and Word Viewer programs included on this CD to view the documents. To use these programs, navigate to the "Viewers" folder on the CD-ROM and double-click the *ppview97.exe* file for PowerPoint Viewer and *wd97vwr32.exe* for Word Viewer.

This program requires that you have the Indeo 5 video codec installed on your computer in order to play the videos. Most systems will have this codec installed. If a valid Indeo 5 driver is not installed, you will not be able to view the videos in the program.

For your convenience, we have included the Indeo drivers installation program on this CD-ROM. To install, simply run the file "iv5setup.exe" located in the "Viewers" folder on this CD-ROM and follow the on-screen instructions. You will need to restart your system after the installation and before running the program.

Launch Instructions for: The Brain and Sensory Plasticity: Language Acquisition and Hearing

1. Insert the disk into the CD-ROM drive. *The Brain and Sensory Plasticity* program should begin automatically. If it does not, go to step 2.
2. Double-click on your My Computer icon on the desktop, then double-click on the CD-ROM icon labeled "Berlin."
3. Open the folder labeled "Berlin" and double-click the *berlin.exe* file to start the program.